HIV PREVENTION AND BISEXUAL REALITIES

Why is there so little HIV education at present directed towards bisexual men and women? This book offers a critical analysis of the issues in public health research and education that prevent adequate attention from being paid to bisexual realities. Addressing the implications of such limited knowledge, the authors raise important questions about the weaknesses of our current response to the HIV/AIDS pandemic.

Through interviews with a variety of bisexual men and women, *HIV Prevention and Bisexual Realities* uncovers innovative, important directions to consider for more effective HIV prevention strategies. The authors' epistemological and methodological assessments of the current state of HIV/AIDS education will be indispensable for community health educators, policymakers, and those who study or work in public health.

VIVIANE NAMASTE is Concordia University Research Chair in HIV/AIDS and Sexual Health and a professor in the Simone de Beauvoir Institute at Concordia University.

TAMARA VUKOV, NADA SAGHIE, ROBIN WILLIAMSON, JACKY VALLÉE, M. LAFRENIÈRE, M. LEROUX, ANDRÉA MONETTE, and JOSEPH JEAN-GILLES are researchers and activists involved in a community advisory committee associated with the research for this book known as Projet Polyvalence (www.polyvalence.ca).

HIV Prevention and Bisexual Realities

VIVIANE NAMASTE, TAMARA VUKOV,
NADA SAGHIE, ROBIN WILLIAMSON,
JACKY VALLÉE, M. LAFRENIÈRE, M. LEROUX,
ANDRÉA MONETTE, JOSEPH JEAN-GILLES

UNIVERSITY OF TORONTO PRESS
Toronto Buffalo London

ISBN 978-0-8020-9993-8 (cloth)
ISBN 978-0-8020-9717-0 (paper)

Printed on acid-free, 100% post-consumer recycled paper with vegetable-based inks.

Library and Archives Canada Cataloguing in Publication

HIV prevention and bisexual realities / Viviane Namaste . . . [et al.].

Includes bibliographical references.
ISBN 978-0-8020-9993-8 (bound). – ISBN 978-0-8020-9717-0 (pbk.)

1. HIV infections – Canada – Prevention.   2. AIDS (Disease) – Canada –
Prevention.   3. Bisexuals – Health and hygiene – Canada.   I. Namaste,
Viviane K.

RA643.86.C3H57 2012   614.5'9939200971   C2012-905141-1

This book has been published with the help of a grant from the Canadian
Federation for the Humanities and Social Sciences, through the Awards
to Scholarly Publications Program, using funds provided by the Social
Sciences and Humanities Research Council of Canada.

The research is supported by the Social Sciences and Humanities Research
Council of Canada (Standard Grant) as well as Concordia University.

University of Toronto Press acknowledges the financial assistance to its
publishing program of the Canada Council for the Arts and the Ontario
Arts Council.

    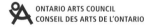

University of Toronto Press acknowledges the financial support of the
Government of Canada through the Canada Book Fund for its publishing
activities.

Contents

List of Illustrations

HIV PREVENTION AND BISEXUAL REALITIES

Introduction

Das HI-Virus hat viele Gesichter. Die Forschung auch. (The HIV virus has many faces. So does research.)

> – Kompetenznetz HIV/AIDS

HIV/AIDS is one of the most important public health issues in contemporary times. It is estimated that over 33 million people are infected with HIV worldwide (UNAIDS 2010), and the numbers continue to increase each year. The gravity of this disease – for individuals, communities, nations, and indeed the entire globe – has required a deep, concerted effort to respond to the many issues raised.

Prevention education occupies an important place in any response to HIV/AIDS. Indeed, reducing the numbers of infections demands both that people understand how HIV is transmitted and that they take the necessary precautions in their behaviour. This task, of course, is not an easy one. This book considers a singular aspect of this challenge, through an examination of prevention education in Québec.

We focus on one facet of HIV prevention – that directed to people who are sexually involved with both men and women. Since HIV is a virus that can be transmitted through unprotected sexual relations, what kinds of educational materials are available to people who have sexual partners of both sexes? As soon as one asks this question, one is confronted with a dilemma. Indeed, although HIV is transmitted through sexual relations, it is extraordinarily difficult to find information that is directed explicitly to people who have sexual relations with *both* men and women. With the notable exception of resources created as a result of this project (presented in chapter 7), a search of Canadian HIV prevention materials housed at the Canadian AIDS Treatment Information Exchange yields no results on education for bisexuals. More than thirty years into an epidemic, there is a virtual absence of posters, pamphlets, videos, or resources targeted specifically to bisexual men and women in Canada.

This absence raises additional questions. How is it that people who are involved with both men and women have been overlooked? What can this gap tell us about our collective response to HIV/AIDS? How do decisions about HIV education get made – the message to send, the populations to reach, the places to distribute materials? Who is involved in the work of education? How do specific campaigns get funded?

This project takes up the challenge of answering these questions. Our work has a number of goals. In the first instance, we seek to document the absence of HIV education specific to bisexuals in Canada. Within Canada and Québec, there has been no large-scale empirical study that focuses on the prevention needs of bisexual men and women.[1] Our research fills a gap in the scientific literature. Yet we seek to do more than simply document an absence in education. Throughout this research, we aim to explain how and why people who have sexual relations with both men and women have been overlooked. Such explanation requires that we move beyond mere description of the problem – for instance, noting the lack of education in this area. Rather, we need to consider some of the perhaps invisible ways in which certain realities and communities have been disregarded. This analysis necessarily takes us into a study of institutions, and as such we examine some of the perhaps invisible workings of HIV/AIDS bureaucracy in Canada. Our study reflects on the kinds of research that informs HIV/AIDS policy, as well as the types of inquiry that are ignored. We consider how policies are translated into concrete administrative procedures, and the ways in which such procedures recognize only certain kinds of communities and populations as affected by the epidemic. This reflection on institutions helps us to explain how and why there is an absence of HIV education for men and women who have sexual relations with both sexes. Finally, in addition to these two goals, our project seeks to intervene in the current situation. After speaking with everyday bisexual men and women about what kinds of education they need, we include an action component in our research – the development of educational materials that are adapted to their realities.

A few words on the authors – this 'we' – are in order. We have come together as a community to address the lack of HIV education for people who have sex with both men and women. Some of us have experience working in HIV/AIDS, and some of us have been involved in community organizing with regards to sexuality. Some of us are academics and make our livings within the university. Others of us have no particular affiliation to university life in its usual incarnation. All of us are committed to asking, and answering, the questions outlined above. Since 2002, we have been working together, as a community-based advisory committee, to conduct this research.

The questions that we have posed above are instructive as we think about HIV education and its limits. Indeed, we begin our inquiry with the remark that there is an absence of appropriate information and materials. To state the matter another way, we start with what is *not* known about HIV education. The question of knowledge, then, is central to our endeavour: we examine how certain gaps in knowledge are perpetuated in HIV/AIDS research, policy, education, and services. And importantly, we seek to produce a different kind of knowledge, one more useful for bisexual men and women. We do so in two ways: by asking bisexual men and women what kind of HIV education they need, and by creating such prevention materials.

These reflections on knowledge – the limits of existing knowledge, the kinds of knowledge that people need to have, the challenge of producing such knowledge as popular education – demand critical analysis of the ways in which research, policy, and education intersect. The different chapters in this book offer detailed examination of how this functions, in order for us to understand more clearly how people like bisexual men and women remain beyond consideration within HIV/AIDS education.

We begin with an overview of mainstream public health research and epidemiology on HIV/AIDS. Here, we introduce the main objectives of such perspectives: to provide an overview of the prevalence of disease within particular populations across time. Yet we also consider some of the limits of mainstream epidemiology and how this research can actually prevent us from understanding the complexity of people's realities. With specific regard to bisexualities, we analyse the ways in which researchers make bisexual men and women disappear in the coding of their data. Part of the reason that we do not have any educational materials adapted to bisexual men and women in Canada is that the research upon which prevention programs are based has underestimated or even effaced bisexual realities.

In chapter 2, we turn our attention to the institutional aspects of HIV/AIDS policy and funding. We examine a key strategic planning document, *Leading Together* (CPHA 2005), which bills itself as a blueprint for action on HIV/AIDS. This document provides an overview of the situation and sets out ambitious targets for action. Our reading of it considers the ways in which bisexuality is ignored within the text. Paradoxically, while specific concerns relevant to bisexual men and women remain unaddressed in *Leading Together*, the document reinforces stigma and discrimination against bisexual men by framing them within the terms of a 'risk group.' The analysis of institutions that we offer explores the ways in which documents like *Leading Together* are central in organizing a collective response to the epidemic. Since the needs of bisexual men and women are ignored therein, it logically follows that there is an absence of prevention initiatives targeted to these realities.

Our reflections on institutions also examine which communities and actors are recognized. We underline the complicated relations between community organizations and the state within a context of neoliberalism and explain the manner in which only state-funded agencies are given a voice and expert status for action in HIV/AIDS research, policy, and education. Since state-funded HIV/AIDS agencies have done a relatively poor job of addressing the needs of bisexual men and women in Canada, this means in effect that bisexual men and women remain excluded, since the organizations and key stakeholders consulted in HIV/AIDS initiatives have little (if any) expertise in bisexualities. Our institutional analysis, then, helps us reflect on who counts as 'community' and on how invisible populations like bisexual men and women are unrecognizable in institutional life.

While chapters 1 and 2 outline some of the profound limits of our knowledge of HIV with regard to bisexual men and women, chapter 3 proposes a methodology for producing a different kind of knowledge. Given that people who have sexual relations with both men and women are regularly ignored in HIV/AIDS research, policy, and education, we design a way of doing research that includes their voices. Moreover, while much of the social science and epidemiological research in HIV/AIDS limits itself to people's behaviour, we focus on their information needs. We ask everyday people about the kinds of prevention they need and how it should be delivered. Having gathered such data, we then developed educational materials that our participants identified as relevant.

Chapter 4 provides an overview of the main results of our study. It examines the problems people have in accessing HIV/AIDS information, as well as in evaluating it. Participants tell us about the ways that existing campaigns do not give them the information they need to protect themselves, and they suggest specific content to include. The reflections offered by our participants also indicate how HIV education should be oriented – its general tone and frame – as well as the importance of distributing it in the mainstream. The results of our empirical research examined in this chapter are contrasted with the knowledge of HIV education presented earlier.

Chapter 5 continues to discuss the empirical data we have gathered, with a specific focus on the needs of women. Drawing on our interviews, we examine the ways in which HIV and STD education is implicitly gendered – for example, the neglect of female partners of bisexual men, the lack of education directed to heterosexual women, or the complete absence of information about woman-to-woman transmission of HIV and STDs. Here again, our data are read alongside broader considerations of existing research and policy in the field: our interviews help us understand how mainstream epidemiology on HIV and STDs excludes women and how this is further manifest in community-based education.

Chapter 6 extends the presentation of data offered. While chapters 4 and 5 outline the specific needs of the people we interviewed with regard to information, this chapter considers the importance of linking HIV/ AIDS *education* to HIV/AIDS *services* more generally. Drawing on our empirical data, we demonstrate that, when it comes to sexual health, people often access information when they need specific services. Since this chapter outlines the importance of access to health care, we also consider some of the main barriers that bisexual men and women face in trying to get services. We give particular attention to the ways in which bisexual women and swingers (couples involved in a stable relationship but who exchange sexual partners) do not have access to relevant information and primary prevention materials. Finally, we consider some of the ways to link education and services, as proposed by our interviewees.

Chapter 7 takes up the challenge of translating our research findings into concrete action. If the men and women we interview provide ample documentation of how their needs are overlooked in health information and services, how can we develop educational materials otherwise? What message should be sent, how should we frame a campaign, how can we link education to services, and where might we want to place the materials we develop? This chapter presents the specific posters that we developed and examines how they attempt to fill the gaps in information and services identified by our participants.

Before we turn to the next chapter, we would like to offer some reflection on the possible different readers who may be interested in our research. As outlined above, this project is situated at the crossroads of a number of different fields: public health, studies in sexuality, empirical sociology, and action research. Students, teachers, and researchers coming from these different traditions will surely recognize the terms of the debates presented. Epidemiologists will understand the ways in which surveillance data inform social policy in the domain of HIV prevention and services. Qualitative researchers in sociology will be interested in the conduct and results of our interviews – the questions we asked, as well as the results obtained. Those within the field of sexuality studies will find here some critical reflections on how sexuality itself is conceptualized – indeed, our study offers the first large-scale empirical study of bisexual men and women within a Canadian context, and as such provides a wealth of data for those interested in thinking about sexuality. And scholars working within the tradition of participatory action research will be able to consider the ways in which the current project involves more than simple commentary on an issue, proposing some concrete strategies to intervene in the social relations we examine. If this book will appeal to these readers in particular (as well as those we have not mentioned here), we are also aware that different kinds of readers may find the current analysis limited insofar as it moves beyond and across traditional fields of academic inquiry. For example, scholars within sexuality studies may desire to see a more developed discussion of identity, given some of the empirical results presented – a preoccupation that is certainly worthy of scholarly investigation, but not the primary focus of this book. Or to take another example, experts in social policy reading this book may wish for a more extended discussion of the relation between epidemiological data and the development of social policy. While we certainly cover this topic, our work does not limit itself to the scholarly debates on social policy and its formulation. We acknowledge the limitations of the present work and the difficulties in bringing together fields of inquiry that often remain distinct (epidemiology, sexuality studies, sociology, action research). Although it remains improbable that all readers will be satisfied completely, we hope that the current research does ask new questions and convinces readers of the need to develop innovative paradigms of inquiry. We suggest that readers approach this book with an appreciation for our attempt to think about HIV education differently.

The questions we pose – and some of the answers that we provide – are, in many ways, outside the box of most mainstream research, policy, and community education on HIV/AIDS. We see this as one of the strengths of our work: we have some critical questions to ask about how and why HIV education has not addressed certain communities more than thirty years into an epidemic. While much of what we have to say is specific to the situation of bisexual men and women, our research also provides an occasion to rethink HIV prevention more generally. Indeed, if rates of HIV transmission continue to rise in the Canadian context – and epidemiological data certainly support this statement (ASPC 2006; SLITSS 2005) – then some critical reflection on the limits and blind spots of HIV education is in order. Our research is to be read in this regard, then: an opportunity to learn how and why different communities have yet to be recognized in HIV education in Canada, and an occasion to act concretely on such inadequacies.

1 The Epistemology of Epidemiology: Understanding the Knowledge and Limits of Public Health Research and Education

We will consistently fail to observe what we do not seek to find.

– H. Burrage

In order to explain the lack of concrete HIV education for people who have sexual relations with both men and women, it is necessary to think critically about the forms of knowledge currently in place about HIV/AIDS. A critical analysis of these epistemological questions – how we know what we know – can provide insight into the response to HIV/AIDS offered so far.

Within the field of public health, the domain known as epidemiology is central. In broad terms, epidemiology seeks to track the presence of disease within a particular population over time. It documents the presence of a specific disease or agent (such as a virus) that causes a disease. Furthermore, epidemiology analyses how a particular disease progresses. Two concepts are central to epidemiology: *prevalence* and *incidence*. The notion of *prevalence* refers to the number of people in a given population who are living with a particular disease. If, for example, seven out of ten Aboriginal people in Montréal have been treated at a hospital or community clinic for tuberculosis, then the TB seroprevalence rate for urban Aboriginal people in Montréal is a staggeringly high 70 per cent. The concept of *incidence* complements that of prevalence and inquires about how many new infections of a specific disease occur within a specific time and population. To take another hypothetical example, an example of HIV incidence would be the recording during one year in Vancouver of ninety-five new HIV infections among intravenous drug users. Incidence tells us how many people have been newly exposed to a particular agent or disease in a select time and place.

The notions of prevalence and incidence are central to the work of epidemiology, and to the field of public health more broadly. Indeed, knowing how many people in a community are living with syphilis, for example, can help us to understand the magnitude of the situation. Similarly, detailed recording of the incidence of hepatitis C can help public health professionals plan their education and services appropriately. Both prevalence and incidence of disease offer a snapshot of the current situation; these notions document how many people are affected and how many new people are affected each year. Yet epidemiology does more than just record this information. Indeed, these data are used predictively by public health: that is to say, they determine where to allocate resources for education and services. Like many government departments, the resources made available to public health are limited. Epidemiology is useful, then, because it can help to trace where a specific disease is most present (based on prevalence and incidence) and where it is likely to increase (based on incidence in particular). If HIV is seen commonly transmitted within the Chinese community of Toronto – and more commonly so than in other ethnocultural communities of similar size in that same city – this information can help public health to allocate specific resources for community-based education and services for this population. Epidemiology is central, then, to public health planning.

Extending from this general introduction to epidemiology, it is important to underline three specific consequences of this framework, particularly when one is discussing HIV/AIDS.

Epidemiology as Informing Social Science Research

The first corollary of an epidemiological paradigm is that this kind of surveillance data is generally used to inform much social science research on HIV/AIDS. Epidemiologists provide a large snapshot of a disease such as HIV/AIDS – for instance, demonstrating its tenacious hold in urban gay male communities. In recent Canadian data, for example, it is stated that 58 per cent of infections are to be found among men who have sexual relations with men (PHAC 2005). In themselves, these data are important, but they do not tell us why these men are not having safe sexual relations or using drugs in a manner that does not transmit blood-borne diseases. Enter the social scientists, who develop both quantitative and qualitative studies that seek to understand more clearly the specific factors that increase risky behaviours with regards to sex and drug use. The data they generate supplement those offered by epidemiology and help to refine more clearly the specific content and approach of HIV education and services. On the level of both research methods and epistemology, it is important to understand here that such social scientific inquiry is determined by epidemiology (Gould 1993). The descriptive data offered in large epidemiological studies direct social scientists' attention to particular communities upon which further research should be conducted. Within such a logic – for example, when HIV seroprevalence rates are seen to be particularly high among certain communities, such as urban gay men – social scientists concentrate on these communities in their own investigations. Certain populations achieve recognition, and priority status within a research agenda, based on epidemiological findings.

Behaviour: Limited as a Basis for Knowledge and Education

This overview of both epidemiological and social scientific research on HIV/AIDS highlights a second issue to keep in mind about such paradigms: these methodologies base themselves primarily on the behaviour of individuals, and by extension, populations. Epidemiologists seek to track the prevalence and incidence of disease within a particular population, and they generally include questions on the sexual behaviour of population members when researching HIV/AIDS (Trostle 2005). Social scientists delve further into this logic, asking in particular about the motivations and context that facilitate people adopting high-risk behaviours, such as sharing needles or unprotected sexual relations (Gould 1993). In both frameworks, the question of behaviour is central, at the level of individuals (what does a person do) as well as the more abstract level of populations (what do a number of people in a particular group, or all of them, do).

While inquiry into behaviour is important and can generate useful knowledge, limitations of this framework remain. In the first instance, studies that focus on the behaviour of people, or populations, conceptualize the problem primarily at the individual level – which is to say, it is about the activity in which an individual engages, and/or the practices common to members of a population. This focus on the individual neglects some of the larger, socio-economic factors that need to be addressed when considering disease. James Trostle provides a useful example of such a weakness in public health approaches that concentrate on modifying the behaviour of individuals, discussing in particular the case of cholera in Ecuador. Cholera is an infectious disease caused by a bacterium, *Vibrio cholera*, which is transmitted in water, food, and (more rarely) faeces. It can cause profound dehydration, dizziness, dulled consciousness, vomiting, and diarrhoea. If untreated, cholera can also cause death. Trostle documents the resurgence of cholera in Latin American since the early 1990s, as well as specific government attempts to prevent its spread. Among such initiatives, Trostle cites the Ecuadorian government slogan on billboards across Quito: 'Lavar las manos es amor en los tiempos del cólera' (Hand-washing is love in the time of cholera). The slogan appeals to the title of a novel by popular Latin American writer Gabriel García Márquez, *Love in the Time of Cholera* (Trostle 2005, 111). This prevention message seeks to modify the behaviour of individuals as a way to reduce transmission of infectious disease. Yet Trostle argues that such a strategy neglects to consider some of the broader political, economic, and social factors that explain how and why individuals – and indeed, certain populations entirely – are especially vulnerable to infectious diseases like cholera. Indeed, in the case of Latin America, the question of safe, regular access to potable water is central. Most poor people do not have such access and are thus at increased risk of exposure to cholera and other diseases transmitted through water. Trostle cites some critical Latin American scholars who explain that poverty is central to understanding the causes of cholera, especially within poor populations (111). The political challenge is not to intervene on the level of behaviour modification of individuals, but rather to attack and transform the root cause of the issue: access to clean water for all. Public health education that limits itself to matters of individual behaviour, then, misses a crucial opportunity to influence policy and social context in order to change the social, political, and economic factors that facilitate the transmission of infectious disease.

Studies concerned with behaviour modification confront an additional challenge, in understanding the connection between people's knowledge of the risks of a particular behaviour and their decision to engage in such behaviour. Studies in HIV/AIDS reveal that, within many communities greatly affected by HIV, members are generally aware of the risks involved in unprotected sexual relations (Massé 1995; PHAC 2005; Trostle 2005). Yet that does not prevent (some) people from engaging in high-risk activities. The provision of information about what activities can transmit HIV is insufficient to alter people's behaviour in this regard. The challenge – at the levels of research, policy, education, and services – is to understand not merely the presence of risk factors, but the underlying causes that facilitate the adoption of risky behaviour: 'Epidemiologists ... sometimes appear to assume that the design of effective interventions depends most heavily on accurately identifying risk factors. But communication theorist Robert Hornik, who was involved in community studies to reduce heart disease, has argued that data on risk factors themselves are insufficient to design effective intervention campaigns. Instead, Hornik contends, one needs to know the risks for the risk factors in order to design interventions that will influence those underlying causes (Hornik 1990, personal communication). For example, knowledge that saturated fats are a strong dietary risk factor for heart disease must be combined with knowledge about why people consume saturated fats' (Trostle 2005, 127). This quotation underlines the importance of investigating health with regards to the underlying causes of health disparities, inequalities, and vulnerabilities to illness. Analysis that simply offers an inventory of the presence of risk behaviours, and interventions that focus exclusively on questions of behaviour modification, miss crucial opportunities to develop complex responses to disease. Perhaps more damningly, such initiatives do little to intervene in the causal factors that explain the reason for ill health and transmission of infectious disease. Importantly, this insight suggests the valuable contributions that disciplines like communication studies can make to public health.

One final issue needs to be addressed with regards to a reliance on behaviour within epidemiological and social scientific studies, particularly in relation to HIV/AIDS. Research that focuses on the risky behaviours of people vis-à-vis HIV necessarily demands that questionnaires and interviews probe into the intimate details of people's lives. In order to determine if people have put themselves at risk for HIV, for instance, one needs to ask sensitive questions about drug use and sexual activity. Social scientists, of course, are trained in how best to conduct research on sensitive topics – from access to the field, to establishing rapport with an interviewee, to conducting an interview (Lee 1993). Nevertheless, studies that gather data on sexual and drug-use behaviour require that participants be comfortable in speaking about their sexuality and drug use, at least within the confines of a research situation. While certainly many individuals are at ease in providing such information, others may be reluctant to participate. In this light, there is an implicit sample bias in most of the social scientific investigations of HIV/AIDS that focus on behaviour: people who choose to participate are already comfortable providing information about their intimate lives and behaviour. But those who are shy, or who would not want to share information about their sexual lives (even within an anonymous survey), will elect not to participate. The limitations of this sample bias are significant: since most of the social scientific research we have on HIV/AIDS in Canada is behaviour-based, this means that we have large amounts of data from people who have no reservations about openly sharing information on their behaviours. But we lack empirical data from individuals who are not comfortable telling researchers about what they do in bed, or the drugs they use. (We expand on these questions with regards to our own research in chapter 3 on methodology.) The absence of data from people who might be reluctant to talk openly about their sex lives and drug use should give us critical pause, especially working in the field of HIV: do individuals who do not share such information adopt high-risk behaviours? Are they *more* at risk than participants who choose to answer surveys, fill out questionnaires, or give interviews? Our inability to answer these questions is a useful reminder of the sample bias in research, which is itself organized through a logic of behaviour-based inquiry. Furthermore, such a sample bias highlights that, while we know a lot about HIV/AIDS and people's behaviour, there are many things we do not yet understand. These methodological limits underline the importance of humility in doing research.

Evidence-Based Medicine and HIV Education

The third corollary that emerges from epidemiology as a perspective is that there is a reciprocal relation between epidemiological studies and the provision of education and services. High rates of HIV seroprevalence and incidence are central to justifying the funding of community groups: these data are used as the evidence necessary for programming and services. Indeed, in the current context, public health appeals to the notion of 'evidence-based medicine' (EBM) as the paradigm to be adopted (Mykalovsky and Weir 2004). EBM implies that decisions about health policy, and the funding of specific programs and initiatives, are grounded in solid empirical data. Health planners fund specific projects or educational campaigns, because scientific studies have demonstrated the impact of disease within certain populations, as well as the response needed to curtail the impact of such disease. Epidemiology is fundamental to establishing the evidence of HIV/AIDS in a specific population, and thus of being able to respond at the level of education and services.

As a paradigm, then, epidemiology occupies an important place in a collective response to HIV/AIDS. The data it generates are surely important and worthwhile. Recent Canadian statistics, for instance, illustrate the fact that HIV continues to be transmitted across the country (ASPC 2006). Moreover, these data tell us something about specific communities that are especially affected by HIV: most HIV infections are located among men who have sex with men in Canada (58 per cent), although there are notably high rates among Aboriginal people (5–8 per cent of all prevalent infections, despite the fact that Aboriginal people comprise only 3.3 per cent of the Canadian population), injection drug users (30 per cent), as well as among people from countries where HIV is endemic (7–10 per cent of all prevalent infections) and prisoners (PHAC 2005). If HIV exists across the country, it is nonetheless especially remarkable within certain populations. Understanding these variations is important in order to address the challenges brought by HIV/AIDS.

Yet epidemiology, like all scientific paradigms, has it limits. And while it is necessary to attend to the lessons raised by epidemiology – information about the sharp rise in HIV infections within a specific population, for example – it is equally imperative to comprehend how the limits of epidemiology prevent us from responding adequately to HIV/AIDS as a scientific and social phenomenon. In this regard, some critical attention to the limits of epidemiology is in order.

One of the most important limits of relying on epidemiology concerns the broader context in which information is to be understood. Here, the limit is not so much with epidemiology per se, as with the contextual information that accompanies it – or not, as the case may be. Some examples will help to illustrate the importance of exercising caution when interpreting epidemiological information. The first example concerns the situation of people from ethnocultural communities. In the first instance, data in Canada and Québec need to be interpreted with caution, as many provincial surveillance systems do not include information on race/ethnicity within the statistics collected (PHAC 2005). Two of the largest provinces, Québec and Ontario, each with large populations of HIV-positive people as well as large immigrant and ethnocultural communities, have not gathered this information until recently – an absence that leads activists to agitate for the inclusion of such categories within epidemiological and surveillance studies.

Within the Canadian context, an important policy change in HIV occurred in 2001 when Immigration Canada required an HIV antibody test of all refugee and asylum claimants.[1] This policy change transformed the visibility of HIV within Canada, as many refugee claimants learned that they, and/or their children, were HIV-positive upon arrival here. This information is necessary to understand available data on people from ethnocultural communities in Canada, some of whom are newly arrived immigrants and refugees. The policy change at Immigration Canada means that we now have more data available on actual numbers of HIV-positive people amongst those coming to Canada. We simply do not have accurate information on HIV rates within ethnocultural communities prior to 2000 (and arguably, even after 2000 – see PHAC 2005). The point to be underlined here is that interpreting epidemiological data requires a broader knowledge of HIV policy and surveillance practices.

A second example illustrates the importance of attending to policy and social context when analysing epidemiological data. Within the available data on HIV rates in ethnocultural communities, the most recent studies show that, proportionally, there are more women than men among the HIV-positive people (Remis and Merid 2004). This information is useful and important, notably in making the argument for education and services adapted to women's realities (Tharao, Massaquoi, and Teclom 2006). Yet here again, surveillance data tell us something about certain populations in particular. In the case of women, it is important to note that provinces such as Ontario and Québec have recently introduced provincial screening programs of all pregnant women (Tharao, Massaquoi, and Teclom). This means, of course, that we have more information about women than men. So one cannot easily conclude from existing epidemiological data that HIV affects women in greater numbers than it does men: that indeed may be the case, but it is difficult – if not impossible – to determine, when we do not have comparable state surveillance data on men. Again, how one interprets epidemiological data ought to account for its broader political, social, and policy context. Understanding such circumstances provides the necessary background to understand how and why certain populations – such as pregnant women, intravenous drug users, and/ or immigrants – are figured worthy of surveillance and study in the first place. This does not mean that HIV does not exist – or indeed is not rampant – in populations outside those recognized in and through state research.

One important limit of epidemiological research, then, is how the statistics presented do or do not account for the social context in question. What the numbers mean, and the political priorities they determine in kind, are themselves produced by specific historical, policy, and social factors (Pisani 2008). A second limitation of epidemiological studies is the descriptive ability of the field itself. Like many scientific approaches, epidemiology relies on particular categories in order to offer a portrait of a disease. In the case of HIV, epidemiology considers the extent to which HIV is generalized across a wide population, as well as where it is located within specific communities and sub-populations. As discussed above, there is an inherent logic to this approach that seeks to identify those communities where HIV is most present in order to fund appropriate education and services. But this approach assumes that one can isolate different communities or sub-populations from one another. Within the field of HIV, for instance, epidemiological categories historically invoked 'high-risk' groups: gay men, intravenous drug users, prisoners (Patton 2002; Shilts 1987). Tracking HIV in these groups was an effort designed to understand the impact of the disease in such populations. The problem – from the point of view of research, policy, education, and services – is that such populations are not always so discreetly organized. Where does one record an HIV infection of an individual who is an urban Aboriginal man who injects cocaine intravenously? Is this type of infection – the cause of which may be unknown – to be considered part of an intravenous drug user (IDU) category, or to be located within the category associated with Aboriginal people? This problem is one causally related to epidemiology itself, insofar as the field depends on classifying individuals into discreet entities whose behaviour can be readily observed and recorded by epidemiologists and social scientists (Pisani 2008).

These difficulties of classification have been evident in the HIV/AIDS epidemic for a long time. Paula Treichler's (1988) compelling argument shows how historically, epidemiological categories locate cases of HIV transmission as caused through heterosexual sex only when other risk factors – homosexual relations, intravenous drug use – have been excluded as possibilities. This logic establishes a hierarchy of mechanisms of transmission. Furthermore, it underestimates the impact of HIV on women in particular. Treichler explains that the world is much more complicated than the neat classifications offered by epidemiological perspectives on HIV. Some gay men also inject drugs, some women who are partners of drug users both share drugs with their lovers and have unprotected sexual relations with them. Accounting for the causal nature of such HIV infection is difficult, if not impossible, within a classificatory logic of distinct categories and populations. The world – perhaps especially our sex lives and drug use – is messier than the tidy formulae and boxes offered by epidemiologists to track disease (Pisani 2008).

The work of epidemiological surveillance, reliant as it is on distinct categories, does more than merely record a factual 'reality' neutrally observed by scientists. Indeed, epidemiology and its categories actually constitute the social world itself: the science paints a picture of distinct populations affected by HIV – men who have sex with men (MSM), injection drug users (IDUs), prisoners, women (curiously often invoked in such a general sense, as if all women were vulnerable to HIV in the same ways). The construction of such distinct populations is then used by public health planners for prevention programs and services. In this manner, epidemiological categories are taken up in everyday institutional life, and their validity further secured. They become the sine qua non of public health. A more detailed exposition of how epidemiological categories and populations are deployed in public health initiatives is presented in the next chapter. For the purposes of our present discussion, it is to be noted that the reification of distinct populations, achieved through the invocation of epidemiological categories, determines the kinds of programs and services that are available in our response to HIV. The separation of complex realities into specific categories curtails our understandings of the nuances of HIV transmission, and therefore how best we can act upon it (Pisani 2008). If a particular population has not been recognized within the terms of epidemiology, it is difficult indeed to secure resources that are adapted to this population. We will see shortly how important this insight is for understanding the lack of HIV prevention programs that are specifically adapted to the needs of individuals who have sexual relations with men and women.

The Cultural Construction of Epidemiological Categories

We have considered the centrality of epidemiology to our understanding of HIV/AIDS, as well as how the limits of epidemiology impede a critical response to infectious disease prevention. In particular, we addressed several limits: a lack of attention paid to social policy and social context; lack of historical and comparative data available to accurately determine incidence and prevalence rates; an over-emphasis on individual behaviour in research (both epidemiological and social scientific); and a classification system of epidemiological categories that negates the complexity of people's lives and behaviours, and privileges certain kinds of knowledge over others.

The last subject – the definition of epidemiological categories – warrants further investigation, particularly in light of doing HIV prevention for people who have sexual relations with both men and women. Indeed, a critical review of how epidemiological categories are defined and operationalized can help explain how it is that there is such a dearth of HIV research on the lives of men and women with bisexual practices, as well as the absence of any prevention education directed to them. Our discussion here considers the cultural construction of epidemiological categories in three substantive issues in particular: gender, sexuality, and race. Having outlined the ways in which epidemiological and public health research reflect specific social and cultural values, we can better understand the absence of HIV prevention for individuals who have sexual relations with both men and women.

Epidemiology and Gender: Where Are the Women in Public Health?

The idea that epidemiological categories are culturally constructed has been advanced by many scholars, notably anthropologists (Massé 1995; Trostle 2005). Feminists have also made this claim, showing how the categories of inquiry used in public health reflect a specific gender bias (Inhorn and Whittle 2001). In a critical review of health scholarship, for example, Marcia Inhorn and K. Lisa Whittle argue that there is a systematic anti-feminist bias in epidemiological research on women's health. They contend that the definition of health itself, and public health in particular, still refers to a male norm – exemplified by the very term *women's health* to designate health issues considered to be unique to women: 'Men's experience of health seem to provide the implicit norm against which women's health must be judged' (557). If this way of defining health is problematic in itself, these scholars go on to argue that even the naming of women's health can obscure the complexities of health issues in that it reduces the field to one concerned with reproductive health. They cite the case of cardiovascular disease, killing half a million women in the United States each year. Yet clinical investigations of this disease in the United States involved thousands of men and no women. In this logic, cardiovascular disease is not understood to be a women's issue. The point raised by Inhorn and Whittle is important: how scientists define disease determines what they observe and how they choose to act. When women are outside the very definition of disease itself, it is thus not surprising that they receive little education or services related to disease prevention.

Indeed, the history of HIV/AIDS provides an excellent example in this regard. In its very early years in North America, AIDS was associated with urban gay men (Patton 2002; Shilts 1987). The condition was colloquially referred to as a 'gay cancer,' and its earliest medical nomenclature was that of GRID – gay-related immune deficiency (Shilts). Such a naming, of course, linked the specific medical condition to a particular group – gay men. Importantly, however, this naming also brought with it a gendered conception to the disease: it was understood as something that affected men. Within the early days of the epidemic, such a gendered understanding of the disease extended to clinical definition of the condition itself: in order to qualify for an AIDS diagnosis, individuals would have to manifest specific opportunistic infections (e.g., toxoplasmosis, Karposi's sarcoma). But the infections considered did not account for the differential impact that HIV had in women's bodies: clinical diagnosis of AIDS did not initially include its impact on vaginal infections, for example (Gorna 1996). In this way, women were excluded from the definition of a clinical condition. Given such a gendered bias, it is not surprising that the early days of the AIDS epidemic had few reported cases of women (ACT-UP New York 1990; Gorna 1996).

If the history of HIV/AIDS includes the exclusion of women – from epidemiological statistics, as well as from clinical trials (ACT-UP New York 1990) – current research and education continue to marginalize, neglect, and/or exclude women within the field of sexual health. Critical attention to both research and education in HIV illustrates this problematic.

In recent years, research and education in public health have paid intermittent attention to the issue of bisexuality. More specifically, the bisexual behaviour of men has been the subject of several research studies within public health and HIV/AIDS (Boykin 2004; Gooß 2002; Kennedy and Doll 2001; Medico, Lévy, Otis, Laroche, and Lavoie 2002). Indeed, any public health focus on bisexuality and HIV/STDs has become synonymous with (an often pathologizing and selective) attention to the bisexual practices of men.

Moreover, the field of public health has produced a category of 'men who have sex with men' as a way to designate males who identify as gay and who have sex with other men, as well as men who do not identify as gay or bisexual, but who nonetheless have sexual relations with other men. This category – men who have sex with men, or MSM – has been taken up by policymakers and service providers. Although the effort to include all kinds of men within the prevention efforts of community-based AIDS organizations is commendable, careful consideration of the existing prevention strategies reveals that there is very little consideration of the actual sexual lives of bisexual men (Farajajé-Jones 1995; Gooß 2002; Kennedy and Doll 2001; Namaste 1998). Educational materials directed at 'men who have sex with men,' for instance, speak about the risks involved in having anal or oral sex with a man, but they do not discuss the risks involved in having vaginal, anal, and oral sex with a woman. The sexual activities of these men with women are implicitly ignored. This creates a situation in which women are made responsible for ensuring safe sexual behaviours with their male partners (Honnens 1998). This absence is significant, given that existing research demonstrates that bisexual men engage in high-risk behaviours with their female partners, notably unprotected anal sex (Beeker 1993; Kalichman, Roffman, Picciano, and Bolan 1998; Padian et al. 1987). The sexual relations of MSM with women, as well as women's practices and health concerns in general, are largely erased.[2] Such an approach illustrates the ways in which public health definitions and usages of the categories 'bisexual' or 'men who have sex with men' are implicitly gendered.

If scholarship and community work are limited in the complex realities of men who have sex with both men and women, there are even fewer resources that address the realities and sexual practices of bisexual women (Feldhorst 1998; Gooß 2002; Medico et al. 2002). Community-based AIDS organizations have few if any materials for distribution that address the sexual lives of women who have sex with both men and women (Feldhorst). Public health research and education consider only bisexual men (if inadequately), leaving the realities and educational needs of bisexual women unaddressed.

Yet the scant public health research that has been undertaken on bisexual women, HIV/AIDS, and STDs shows that the risks are not negligible and that many legitimate public health questions remain unaddressed and unanswered (both in health research and the health and information needs of bisexual women). Research shows that bisexual women are at higher risk for both HIV/AIDS and STDs than either exclusively heterosexual women or lesbians (Bailey, Farquhar, Owen, and Mangtani 2004; Bauer and Welles 2001; Bevier, Chiasson, Heffernan, and Castro 1995; Gonzalez et al. 1999; Scheer et al. 2002).

Regarding woman-to-woman transmission, the sparse research that exists documents reported cases of HIV transmission between women (though actual risk remains debated and unknown) and a non-negligible risk of woman-to-woman transmission of STDs (particularly HPV, herpes, and trichomoniasis) (Bauer and Welles 2001; Kwakwa and Ghobrial 2003; Marrazzo, Coffey, and Bingham 2005; Rich, Back, Tuomala, and Kazanjian 1993; Troncosa, Romani, Carranza, Macia, and Masini 1995). Significantly, a recently reported instance of woman-to-woman transmission of HIV in the United States involved a case in which one of the partners was an openly bisexual woman known to be HIV-positive who used protection only with her male partners, as advised by her physician (Kwakwa and Ghobrial).

Importantly, Bauer and Welles (2001) have noted a marked insufficiency of research on non-HIV STDs, which may be more readily transmitted between women than HIV/AIDS. This finding was confirmed by the women in our study, who had many questions and noted a serious lack of information and services in this respect. (We elaborate on these results in chapter 5.) Bauer and Welles's study also found a correspondingly low level of STD/HIV testing among women who have sex with women in proportion to the risk they face, consistent with findings that women who have sex with women are less likely to use health care resources (particularly preventative health care) (Stevens 1992). Marrazzo, Coffey, and Bingham (2005) found that many of the lesbian and bisexual women in their study had a limited awareness of the potential for STD transmission between women and recommend increased STD-focused prevention education that emphasizes the plausibility of STD transmission among women who have sex with women.

Studies have also documented the institutionalized exclusion of women who have sex with women from 'risk group' categories, resulting in the public health and popular perception that sex between women is risk free (Bauer and Welles 2001; Marrazzo, Coffey, and Bingham 2005; Richardson 2000). Furthermore, the scarcity of data on woman-to-woman transmission of HIV/AIDS can be attributed in part to the gendered manner in which a hierarchy of 'risk factors' shapes the way in which transmission between women is epidemiologically substantiated. Sex between women is established as a route for HIV transmission only when all other possible risk factors are eliminated (sex with men, tattoos, piercings, injection drug use, transfusions). In other words, as Kwakwa and Ghobrial (2003) note, the epidemiological precedence that other risk factors are given in establishing HIV acquisition among women who have sex with women may mask the actual risk of transmission via sex between women. These data and the results of our study raise important questions about the epidemiological construction of sexual risk in public health, and how the gendered nature of risk categories and risk factors contributes to the erasure of women.

In all of these ways, then, women are excluded from the terms of epidemiology and public health used to understand disease. To state that epidemiological categories are gendered is to acknowledge the methodological difficulties discussed above in the naming and defining of disease. The next section offers a different illustration of this same problematic, through specific case studies of how sexuality itself is defined within public health research.

Epidemiology and the Erasure of Bisexuality

The cultural construction of epidemiological categories and research, evident in the (lack of) research on women's sexual health, is also realized with respect to sexuality. As noted above, public health research on HIV/AIDS functions with numerous epidemiological classifications. Among these, the category of men who have sex with men (MSM) holds an important place, given the higher rates of HIV seroprevalence within such a population than within the general society. MSM in Québec, for instance, constitute 62.5 per cent of recorded HIV cases for the period 2002–4 (SLITSS/MSSS 2005), while national statistics across Canada indicate that MSM make up 45 per cent of HIV seroprevalence cases for 2005 (ASPC 2006). It is important to underline that these statistics include the realities of men who self-identify as bisexual in health service settings, as well as those who reveal that they have had sexual relations with other men without necessarily naming themselves as gay or bisexual (ASPC 2006; SLITSS/MSSS 2005). Yet how this category is defined and operationalized reveals specific cultural assumptions about sexuality.

The category MSM is at once nebulous and pervasive. Patton (2002) situates its emergence in and around 1989 at the Global Programme on AIDS. The nomenclature was designed to include and reflect a broad range of men who have sex with other men – those who might call themselves bisexual, those who are active in gay male communities, and those who would refuse labels entirely. From the perspective of public health, MSM calls attention to specific behaviour rather than identities (here, we note the centrality of behaviour to public health research on HIV/AIDS once again). Certainly, the effort to cast a wide net and include a multitude of realities is worthwhile indeed. Some gay male activists, however, have critiqued the adoption of MSM as a category, because it erases the particularity of gay men's culture and lives – a phenomenon especially relevant in attending to HIV/AIDS education and services (Lavoie 1998). If MSM risks evacuating the specific impact of HIV on gay men in particular, careful analysis reveals that, despite its goodwill and rhetoric, it actually does very little to gather information about men who live or identify anything other than gay. Indeed, arguably MSM as a category reinforces a specific association between MSM and gay men, eclipsing the lives and needs of men who might call themselves bisexual, or who might not be concerned at all with how they name their sexuality. A specific example taken from Canada context will help to illustrate this point.

The research study in question is known as *The Men's Survey* (Myers, Godin, Calzacara, Lambert, and Locker 1993). Although it is now somewhat dated, it still remains one of the most comprehensive large-scale investigations of MSM populations in Canada. The survey was completed across Canada by 4803 men and focused on gathering information about their knowledge, attitudes, and behaviours (KAP) in relation to HIV. (Here, we can witness again a public health research program that gathers information on behaviour in order to design effective education.) The sheer scope and volume of the survey is impressive in itself. Yet when one examines its methodology closely, one can observe specific difficulties in thinking about sexuality.

Within this study, researchers considered how respondents identify themselves in sexual orientation, as well as their sexual behaviour in the past year. In their coding of the data, however, the researchers required that a respondent have sexual relations with both men and women within the past twelve months in order to be grouped under the category 'bisexual.' Thus, men who identified themselves as bisexual but who had had sexual relations only with men in the past year were re-categorized as 'gay men with a previous heterosexual experience' (Myers et al. 1993, 31–2). In other words, a participant in this survey had to have had sexual relations with both a man and a woman in the past twelve months in order to be considered 'really' bisexual. There is a logic particular to Western cultural assumptions of bisexuality at work here – the idea that bisexuality does not really exist, that in actuality, people are really *more* attracted to women or to men. Critical scholars and activists have analysed the ways in which

Western conceptions of sexuality inscribe bisexuality to be literally impossible (Angelides 2001; Hall and Pramagiorre 1996; Hutchins and Ka'ahumanu 1991; Tucker 1995). One can witness such a conception of bisexuality within the coding of the research team in *The Men's Survey*: it is not enough to say that one is bisexual, it is something that has to be proven. Furthermore, the coding of the data appeals to a specific period: the previous twelve months. Fleeting and evasive, the category 'bisexual' comes with an expiry date. Here, a behaviour-based definition of sexuality reinforces a specific cultural belief that bisexuality is, in itself, unsustainable.

Attention to the coding and analysis of groups other than 'bisexual men' within *The Men's Survey* further reveals how cultural myths and stereotypes inform the definition and use of epidemiological categories in research. This study found that many of the men in the survey who identified as gay had had sexual relations with a woman in the past year – in fact, 30.8 per cent of respondents who labelled themselves 'gay' had had sexual relations with a woman within the previous twelve months (Myers et al. 1993, 32). Yet the researchers did not take this information and recode how these gay men labelled themselves – they did not, for instance, come up with a category of 'heterosexual men with a previous homosexual experience.' The recoding of sexual orientation, in this research, was limited to that of men who labelled themselves bisexual. In a similar manner, while men had to prove their bisexuality through sexual relations with both men and women over the past twelve months, men who named themselves gay had to demonstrate sexual relations with another man at least once in their lives (Myers et al., 32). In others words, a man can (for example) have sex with one male partner twenty years previously and be considered 'gay' for the purposes of the research. Conversely, a bisexual respondent needs to offer proof of relations with both men and women within the past twelve months. Gayness is measured across a lifetime, while bisexuality is only a specific phase. Here again, a behaviour-based definition of bisexuality instantiates particular cultural assumptions of sexuality – that bisexuals have to prove their bisexuality through behaviour, and that indeed, bisexual men are always having sex!

The comparative analysis offered here can help us understand, then, the ways that cultural beliefs and meanings influence how researchers define and use particular categories. At the level of methodology, one of the important lessons to be learned is that there is great inconsistency in how different categories of people are conceptualized, studied, and examined – discrepancies that seriously compromise the possibility of any meaningful generalization from the research results. Research studies like *The Men's Survey* require that a male have sexual relations with both men and women in the past year in order to be classified as bisexual. By definition, such a participant needs to have had at least two sexual partners. In contrast, *The Men's Survey* simply requires a male respondent name himself as gay and have had at least one sexual relation with another man during his lifetime in order to be classified as gay for the purposes of data analysis. Here, then, the coding of data creates differential variables for distinct sub-populations: bisexual men need to have had at least two partners (one of each sex), while gay men can have only one partner. On the level of research methods, it is problematic to compare data from specific variables that have been defined in radically different ways.

The problems with a behaviour-based definition of bisexuality are also evident in some recent data on health issues in Québec. In a national survey on health care, the Québec Office of Statistics included specific information on sexual orientation (ISQ 1998). This is, of course, a welcome initiative: this survey represents one of the first large-scale, probabilistic inquiries on a population that gives attention to sexual health needs. The importance of such information – for future research, policy, education, and services – cannot be underestimated. That said, the survey design relies on a behaviour-based definition of sexuality. In order to be included in the specific data relevant to sexual orientation, respondents had to have been sexually active.

The information presented provides clear evidence that bisexual men and women experience profound marginalization and social isolation, and that attention to their health needs ought to take such a context into consideration. The data suggest that the situation faced by bisexual men and women is more distressing than that faced by other sexual minorities: they experience stronger feelings of isolation, more frequent suicide attempts, and higher consumption of alcohol among bisexual women than among lesbians. Yet the design of the study, like that of *The Men's Survey*, appeals to a behaviour-based definition of sexuality. This means that different subgroups of sexual minorities – lesbians, gay men, and bisexuals – have not been defined in the same way. While lesbians and gay men need to have had one sexual partner in order to be included in these data, bisexuals need to have had two partners – one of each sex. The two groups being compared do not have the same number of required sexual partners.

Attention to the coding and definition of epidemiological categories is important, because codes organize respondents into different groups and sub-populations, such as gay men, bisexual men, 'gay men with a previous heterosexual experience.' These codes, then, determine how information will be grouped, organized, analysed, and presented. If the specific coding of the data reflects cultural assumptions, then these will manifest in the research results themselves (Trostle 2005; Pisani 2008). Our analysis of some of the most widely recognized work on MSM in Canada illustrates the ways in which prejudice, stereotypes, and misinformation are organized in the definition and use of research categories.

One final point to be made here: the manner in which the research team of *The Men's Survey* defined bisexuality has curtailed membership within such a category. Men who called themselves bisexual but who had had sex only with men in the past year were not considered to be bisexual for the data coding. In this regard, the specific definition of the category actually erases the experiences and realities of bisexual men. Paradoxically, then, this kind of research makes it more difficult to see and understand bisexual men (to say nothing of their female partners!). Epidemiological categories like those deployed in *The Men's Survey* literally make some bisexual men disappear. Such erasure reflects a broader social relation in which bisexuality is impossible. Ironically, this effacement of bisexual men – and bisexuality more generally – occurs within a broader context of public health organized under a banner of MSM – a collocation designed supposedly to include men who might identify themselves other than gay. In a similar vein, the Québec health survey excludes all people who call themselves bisexual but who have not been sexually active with both men and women. The data of this survey underestimate bisexuals in general, but perhaps especially bisexual youth, who may or may not have had many sexual partners – regardless of their sex. Like *The Men's Survey*, this research design obscures our understanding of the vast scope of bisexualities. Far from helping us to gain further insight into non-gay men within an MSM population, we believe that many studies in this domain actually obscure our understandings of this issue. Indeed, social and epidemiological research that relies on behaviour-based definitions of sexuality significantly underestimates the very presence of bisexual men and women themselves, since it organizes data only with regard to those who are recently active with both men and women.

These reflections on the literal erasure of bisexuality are important for helping us to understand how cultural meanings inform epidemiological categories. But they can also assist us in explaining the utter lack of HIV education for men and women with bisexual behaviour in Canada. We have argued above that education and services are dependent on research: scientific studies are central to the 'evidence' required by health policy experts and planners. Yet in the case of bisexuality, the available research actually underestimates the very existence of bisexual men and women. Health policymakers and departments of public health across Canada have yet to recognize bisexual realities in any meaningful way, in part because the available scientific research makes this population, and this reality, disappear. It is difficult indeed to provide HIV education for a community, or a reality, that does not exist.

Race and Public Health: Cultural Stereotypes and Epidemiological Research

The third way in which we would like to demonstrate the influence of culture and society on epidemiology is through a consideration of HIV prevention research with respect to matters of race, with particular reference to the situation of MSM. As noted above, MSM emerged as a category that was designed to include all kinds of men, regardless of their identity. Yet how this particular category has come to be taken up in public health research reflects broader ideas about matters of race and ethnicity, and their connection to sexuality.

Within epidemiological and social scientific studies on MSM, researchers regularly make the important distinction between identity and behaviour (Myers et al. 1993). Many offer further reflection on the particular challenges in developing prevention materials for men who do not call themselves 'gay' or 'bisexual,' but who nonetheless have sexual relations with other men. Having acknowledged that there is a difference between identity and behaviour, researchers offer empirical evidence that for many men, having sex with another man is possible, especially if they take a dominant, insertive role in anal intercourse (Gooß 2002). Such a practice does not, according to experts in this domain, challenge these men's heterosexuality or sexual identity. Public health researchers regularly cite anthropological data to support their claim – ethnographic studies that illustrate the centrality of an active/passive status with regard to sexuality, as opposed to a particular name, label, or sexual orientation (see, for instance, Kulick 1998).

These reflections on such realities are intimately connected to questions of culture within both anthropological and public health scholarship. The argument advanced is that researchers and service providers need to attend to cultural differences in this regard: men from Latin America may organize their sexualities primarily through an active/passive distinction, as opposed to a gay/straight divide. Health policy, services, and education, then, need to understand the ways in which culture informs sexuality. Such attention to the relations between culture and sexuality is worthwhile indeed: scholarship in critical public health and ethno-epidemiology in particular has certainly demonstrated the central role that cultural meanings play in determining what services people access, and how they do so (Trostle 2005; Massé 1995). That said, there are accompanying limitations to such an approach.

The first such limitation is related to the sexual behaviours themselves. This kind of research argues for the centrality of an active/passive distinction in questions of anal intercourse. Yet virtually nothing is said about other sexual activities in which non-gay-identified men engage with other men – oral sex, or mutual masturbation, for example. Thus, although analysis of sexuality that does not impose a Western identity-based conception of sexual orientation is important, one must inquire nonetheless whether such a framework will be useful for doing prevention work with the men who do not engage in anal sex at all with other men. Here, then, public health research has organized itself around a specific activity – anal sex – even at the precise moment that it argues for the importance of attending to a diversity of men's sexual realities.

The second limitation of this argument is centrally concerned with culture. An invocation of this active/passive distinction is inevitably linked to *certain* cultures and ethnicities. For example, public health research outlines the importance of such nuance with particular concern for Latin American men. Interestingly – and coincidentally – the specific cultural and ethnic groups named can vary somewhat within different national contexts: researchers in the United States point out the importance of considering culture and MSM with specific reference to Hispanics and black men (Boykin 2004), Canadian researchers refer to black communities in particular (Crichlow 2004), and Australian scholars designate Latin and Arab men as those for whom sexuality with men is conceived through an active/passive frame (Pallota-Chiarolli 1998). The designation of such specific communities in distinct national contexts, of course, reflects in part the visibility and importance of such populations in these locations.

Yet the argument that one must attend to culture in thinking about 'ethnic' men who do not call themselves gay or bisexual, but who still have sexual relations with men, paradoxically assumes that matters of culture are not equally relevant in a consideration of white men in the United States, Anglo-Canadian men, or Anglo-Australian men. This argument, then, figures 'culture' as something that belongs exclusively to the non-white and/or immigrant individual (Bannerji 2000). Having established culture as somehow outside an unmarked white norm, this discourse then goes on to configure its relation to sexuality: a refusal to name oneself 'gay' or 'bisexual' is a product of specific cultural meanings. This argument – while on the surface attentive to matters of diversity – does not consider the white men who also do not choose to label themselves 'gay' or 'bisexual.' Indeed, public health research does not offer extended reflection on the situation of a non-gay-identified white man who elects to have sexual relations with another man – even anal sex, in the 'active' role – in relation to the white man's particular ethnic and cultural background. His sexuality is not explained or examined – with the appropriate supporting anthropological data, of course – as part of his tradition, social context, or ethnic world view. Within public health research, 'culture' is something invoked only when non-white bodies are concerned.

Our argument about these limits highlights some of the issues that public health has chosen not to investigate. Such an attention to what public health does *not* study is further significant in a critical examination of its discourse on ethnicity and MSM. Invocations of the active/passive distinction and the importance of attending to it in culturally sensitive HIV education inevitably refer to certain cultural communities in particular – black American, Latin American, Arab. Discussion of MSM and an active/passive distinction do not, however, regularly refer to Asian communities at all.[2] Could such an absence be explained in part by cultural stereotypes that see Asian men's sexuality as inevitably passive (Fung 1991; Pallota-Chiarolli 1998)? Indeed, can one even imagine a Vietnamese man who calls himself bisexual? A Korean man who has sex with other men, but does not see himself as gay? A concern with matters of culture and ethnicity in sexual health education – while certainly important and worthwhile – can too easily reinforce cultural stereotypes of sexuality and race: the hyper-sexualized black man, the passive Asian, the Arab or Latin stud who will have sex with a man as long as he plays the 'active' role. These stereotypes have in part determined the kinds of questions asked, and answered, in public health.

The definition and operationalization of non-gay-identified men within an MSM category is intimately tied to matters of culture. Within public health research, the sexuality of non-gay men is explained with reference to their ethnicities and cultures when these men are not of an Anglo heritage. Paradoxically, however, there is virtually no analysis of how ethnicity and culture affect the sexualities of men who are white, who do not identify as gay or bisexual, and who have sexual relations with other men. Within public health research on MSM, ethnicity matters when one needs to explain the non-gay MSM who are not white and or immigrants. This discourse demonstrates that white men – be they gay, bisexual, or non-gay identifying – stand as an unmarked norm within public health research. This example provides an additional illustration of the ways in which epidemiological categories are infused with cultural meanings.

Conclusion

In order to understand why there is no HIV education directed to bisexual men and women in Canada, it is necessary to think critically about the kinds of knowledge we have in the field. Our consideration of public health research has demonstrated the centrality of epidemiology to our knowledge and action on infectious disease. Moreover, we have analysed how epidemiology is not a neutral, 'objective' science: specific cultural and social values inform the definition, meaning, and operationalization of epidemiological categories. Such categories are implicitly gendered, excluding women from their terms of reference, and/or significantly underestimating women's risk of infectious disease. The operationalization of epidemiological categories in public health also instantiates specific cultural views on sexuality – demanding that bisexuals prove their sexualities (a requirement not made of other sexualities in the same way), and literally making some men and women who call themselves bisexual disappear from the research. And epidemiology in HIV/AIDS also reinforces specific ideas about race and ethnicity – culture is something to be thought about in relation to immigrant and or non-white bodies, but is not particularly relevant for white bodies. In all of these ways, epidemiology provides a useful illustration of how social and cultural variables determine science and the doing of research.

The consequences of epidemiology and its limits are, of course, significant. Epidemiology functions as the 'evidence' of public health education and services. So when epidemiology makes a particular population disappear, it is not surprising to note the virtual absence of education and services adapted to such a reality. The next chapter examines how this functions in more depth, through a consideration of how public health relies on and appeals to epidemiological evidence in its daily activities. The mundane work of public health systems, organized through epidemiological categories and knowledge, reinforces the misrecognition of people who have sexual relations with both men and women. Analysis of how this occurs at the institutional level can assist us in further understanding how certain populations are absent in HIV education in Canada. The next chapter, then, offers an institutional analysis of HIV education in Canada and considers the ways in which the administrative response to HIV constitutes an erasure of bisexualities.

2 Institutional Ethnography: Understanding the Links between Research, Policy, and Education on HIV/AIDS

When political strategies are grounded in theory – sociological or political – there is a strong tendency for them to misfire, or worse yet, backfire. Grass-roots organizing is better based on a sociology committed to describing how society actually works.

– George Smith

In the previous chapter, we examined the limits of the research that we have on bisexualities and HIV/AIDS. This chapter continues this line of inquiry but extends it to a broader institutional analysis. If research is significant in the fight against HIV/AIDS – and one could hardly deny this point – its importance lies not only in the actual research per se, but in how it is used. The knowledge generated in the field does not, at least in an ideal sense, sit idly on a shelf in some researcher's office. Rather, HIV/AIDS research – and specifically prevention research – is conducted with an eye to develop, implement, and evaluate successful prevention programs. Ultimately, such research is instrumental in helping to reduce the transmission and impact of HIV/AIDS.

But how is research used, exactly? What are the ways in which it is taken up within institutions in order to inform the development of, for example, HIV education and services? How do we understand the link between research and education in a manner more complex than simply stating that a relation is there? What particular theoretical and methodological frameworks could assist us here, and why might they be useful? This chapter addresses these questions. Its aim is to explore how the connections between research and education are formulated in particular institutional locations. Moreover, this chapter makes the argument that we need to understand how such institutions work – how they make use of research to inform education – in order to explain how and why there is a dearth of HIV prevention for men and women with bisexual behaviour, in Canada and elsewhere. While this argument was made with respect to matters of epistemology and methodology in the previous chapter, here we incorporate a specifically institutional analysis in our framework.

Institutional Ethnography

There are, of course, many different approaches one could take in studying institutions within disciplines such as sociology, political science, or economics. We have chosen to focus our attention on one particular framework within the tradition of anglophone sociology: institutional ethnography. We will briefly outline the terms and parameters of institutional ethnography here and then proceed to apply this method to our analysis of HIV education.

Institutional ethnography is associated with the Canadian sociologist Dorothy Smith. In very general terms, institutional ethnography (IE) seeks to explore how people's experience of the everyday social world is structured by larger institutional relations. It begins in the mundane details of everyday life but is also attentive to the broader social, economic, and institutional factors that determine everyday life itself. In this regard, IE offers a model of inquiry that seeks to offer both a micrological and a macrological analysis. IE is heavily influenced by a number of theoretical traditions: Marxism, feminism, ethnomethodology, and phenomenology. It is useful for us to outline them here briefly, in order to provide appropriate background information for the reader.[1] Smith's work began with an avowed commitment to creating knowledge relevant for women's lives. She wanted to create a kind of sociology for women – not an abstract field that either ignored women entirely or objectified them in its analysis. This concern with creating relevant knowledge involves, for Smith, thinking about the everyday. Here she draws on phenomenology, with its emphasis on subjective meanings for people – an exploration of how people see the world and themselves within it. Smith is also heavily influenced by the sociological tradition known as ethnomethodology. Ethnomethodology is a framework that seeks to explain the invisible but central workings of social life, phenomena that are 'seen but unnoticed' (Garfinkel 1967). Resolutely empirical, this tradition uncovers what we take for granted and demonstrates how such taken-for-granted elements are actually fundamental to how the world works – the interactions between people within it, and the meanings they give to certain events. The influence of ethnomethodology in Smith's work is complemented by the Marxist tradition, notably its concept of social relations. For Marx, the proper task of theoretical explanation is to understand how the world is organized so that it can be improved. Objects (or people, or communities) of scientific study are not to be reified as distinct, abstract entities, but are rather to be grounded within the specific social relations in which they are embedded. The Marxist project, of course, privileges the notion of class within this idea of social relations – where people are located in relation to money and capital (do they own the factory, for instance, or must they sell their labour in exchange for a wage?). While a classical Marxist analysis emphasizes class, its concept of a social relation is important. It refers to how particular individuals and groups are situated in relation to each other. The idea of social relations invokes a broader perspective than that of isolated individuals – the social relations of capitalism, for instance, determine how we interact daily: who sells their labour power in exchange for a wage; who owns a factory, makes money, and continues to buy more factories; who bakes bread to sell it, and who relates to them (as well as why and how) when they enter the bakery. Social relations are often invisible phenomena that structure and organize everyday life. Smith uses this idea of social relations, but takes it one step further and advances the notion of 'ruling relations.' Ruling relations, for Smith, refers to the institutional activities that organize the social world. They are coordinated through texts, documents such as policy briefs, and even administrative forms.

These theoretical influences on IE are used in combination by Smith, as well as other practitioners in the field, in order to explain how the world works. It is a framework that draws on the small details of everyday life (the influence of ethnomethodology is clear) as well as a broader social and institutional analysis, which can help put such details into perspective. IE seeks to offer a nuanced understanding of how the world is put together, so that we can think critically about how to change it for the better.

Some specific examples of IE studies will help to illustrate this abstract discussion of IE. The first example is taken from Smith's work herself and concerns elementary school education. She cites the case of a teacher who divides a classroom into several different reading groups: one for students who are relatively skilled at reading, with good vocabulary and reading comprehension; one for students who have average skills in this domain; and a final group for individuals who are not the strongest readers and who may require additional assistance. The experience of individual students in this classroom will be interpreted with regard to their particular time spent in a specific group. But Smith draws our attention to some of the broader social relations at play. Teachers create such groups within a classroom because they cannot possibly assist each child individually within the time allotted to reading: individual accompaniment of thirty or more students in reading would itself take an entire day! So teachers break a large group up into smaller ones and move between them – spending perhaps a little more time with the readers who may require additional assistance if they can, or having a teaching assistant do such work if such resources are available. Smith argues that this decision is not merely a matter of teachers' choice or individual preference. Rather, it reflects a pragmatic strategy to deal with their limited time and resources. In this regard, such an immediate pedagogical choice is itself determined by larger institutional issues – the allocation of resources to a school board and specific school, the number of students deemed to be 'appropriate' in an elementary school class, whether or not a teacher can make use of the services of a teaching auxiliary. Smith brings into focus what is often invisible and helps us to understand how ruling relations affect our everyday experience of the world.

A different example of IE investigation is available in the work of Nancy Naples (2003). She conducted an empirical investigation of mothers on welfare who were also enrolled in post-secondary education. Naples examined the ways in which these women's experience of post-secondary education were determined by the administrative apparatus of state welfare. For example, they were required to have professors sign attendance sheets and provide these to the welfare office, as proof of active involvement in the program. This administrative procedure – designed to ensure money was allocated only to 'deserving' students – compelled these women to divulge their source of income to their professors. Given the negative connotations associated with welfare in the popular mindset, these women felt stigmatized: no other students had to tell their teachers how they paid for school. Moreover, such administrative rules were poorly adapted to the realities of being a mother. If a child was sick, for instance, sometimes mothers would bring the child to class – risking negative judgment from their peers and teachers – rather than miss class, because if they were absent, they would be financially penalized by the welfare office. Naples shows how such administrative procedures in turn determine the choices that mothers in school on welfare can make. Their experience of post-secondary education is one ordered by broader institutional relations.

A third example of an IE will help clarify the approach. This specific example is also closely related to the subject of this book, in that it concerns the question of HIV/AIDS. Scholar George Smith (who worked with Dorothy Smith as a researcher at the Ontario Institute for Studies in Education, but is of no relation) conducted an institutional ethnography of how HIV/AIDS was organized in the province of Ontario in the late 1980s (G. Smith 1995). In his conversations and involvement with activist groups, Smith knew that there were experimental treatments available for people living with HIV/AIDS. However, most of those treatments were unavailable in Ontario at the time. The explanation offered by community leaders was, in Smith's words, a 'speculative account' (22). They invoked the notions of homophobia (AIDS being strongly associated with gay men in the popular imaginary at the time) and/or the idea of bureaucratic red tape. Smith was interested in truly understanding why such treatments were unavailable: was it really because of homophobia, as was so often claimed? He set out to undertake an IE of HIV/AIDS. In addition to his conversations and collaboration with activists, Smith interviewed government bureaucrats and public health officials and consulted key policy documents in this domain. What he found was that experimental treatments were not available for people living with HIV/AIDS in Canada at the time because there was no clear infrastructure to deliver such treatments. Government policies and procedures, notably the approval of experimental drugs at Health Canada, were not equipped to address experimental treatments for HIV/AIDS, and in any event did not move quickly. Smith demonstrates that the government response to the epidemic was focused primarily on palliative care: since the disease was understood to be fatal (a conception disputed by many people living with HIV/AIDS at the time), government resources were allocated to services for the dying. Smith's research in this area is important in a number of ways. In the first place, this kind of inquiry helps people understand what is invisible to them – the government response that is organized exclusively along the lines of palliative care. Such an analysis can then be used by grassroots activists in their own work. Indeed, Smith recounts how this insight focused the activities of activists in lobbying for a treatment infrastructure in Canada. This kind of sociological inquiry, then, is useful in a broader project of social change. Moreover, Smith's work is particularly exemplary of the careful attention that IE pays to the question of knowledge itself. He writes about how everyday people living with HIV/AIDS knew that the condition was not necessarily fatal, and that certain experimental treatments available elsewhere could prolong life and preserve health. At the same time, this insight was not embodied in the knowledge of HIV/AIDS in policy documents or the government response. IE thinks about such a disjuncture, in order to explain how certain forms of knowledge are central to ruling – in this instance, the 'knowledge' that HIV/AIDS was fatal was used to inform government relations that supported palliative care as the primary service response. Smith underlines the centrality of such a disjuncture – what is often termed a 'line of fault' in IE (20) – in defining a research problematic: 'My research began, not in the objective domain of sociological theory, but with everyday events in people's lives, and in their problems of knowing – of being told one thing, but in fact knowing otherwise on the basis of personal experience. Such "ruptures of consciousness" provided a starting point for the research that went on to explicate how a regime works' (21). Institutional ethnography, then, is a project wherein matters of knowledge are central and where one examines the intimate connections between specific forms of knowledge and ruling.

Institutional Ethnography and Research Methods: How to Collect Data

The specific methods in doing an institutional ethnography vary. They can include interviews, analysis of policy documents, and participant observation of relevant sites (Campbell and Gregor 2002). Yet IE does not necessarily limit itself to such strategies and often uses many of these approaches in combination. IE also proposes a new way of thinking about methods – instead of approaching interviews as a site solely to gather data, for example, some researchers use the interview as an occasion to verify their reflections, observations, and tentative explanations about how the world is organized, checking these with and against the perceptions of the people being interviewed (Mykalovskiy and McCoy 2002). IE can also rely on more informal methods of collecting data – conversations with people that occur spontaneously, or a passing remark heard at a rally. These sources of information can be useful (and sometimes extremely significant) points of entry to understanding the organization of the social world. In its methods, IE is less concerned with outlining a recipe for specific ways in which data are to be gathered (Campbell and Gregor; Smith 2005). Rather, it draws on a variety of methodologies and approaches in order to obtain empirical data.

If the field is open to many different kinds and types of methods, we ought also to underline that texts and documents play a central role in many IE projects. In Roxana Ng's (1995) analysis of multiculturalism as ideology, for example, she engages in a detailed examination of the government pronouncement on multiculturalism given by Prime Minister Trudeau in 1971. In a similar manner, Himani Bannerji (1995) looks at the ways in which imperialism has been justified through appeal to certain kinds of knowledge and documents. She shows how James Mill's *The History of British India* was central to British imperial policy in India. Mill's research contends, for instance, that Muslims in India were a particularly aggressive and barbaric people, and Bannerji examines how such a framework is invoked to provide an alibi for colonial rule. In a different example, George Smith (1995) makes his analysis by reading official state documents in the field of health – such as the Health Promotion and Protection Act of Ontario, and state documents related to Canada's Emergency Drug Release Program. Analysis of documents can also focus on the micrological level – as evidenced in Ng's study of immigrant workers and a counselling agency in Toronto. She demonstrates the ways in which the administrative intake forms used by the counsellors structure their relations with the clients, and how these in turn determine the quality of that relation with regards to the mandate of the organization, but not necessarily the complex needs of immigrant women themselves (Ng 1988). In all of these IE studies, and many others not mentioned here, documents are central to helping scholars understand how the world is put together.[2]

Analysis of documents in IE is done with an interest in understanding their relations to ruling. The point is not just to understand the content of a form or a prime minister's speech. The purpose of such an endeavour is to comprehend how the world is organized, and the central role of documents in this regard. When the government announces a new policy on multiculturalism, for instance, the accompanying documents are used to inform policy in a variety of fields – education, history, official languages. Similarly, when state documents on HIV/AIDS services limit themselves to palliative care, they focus the government response to the epidemic in such a manner. Documents, then, are not neutral in themselves – they are taken up and used, they inform future research, policy, and services. They are texts in action, and as such, they constitute social relations (Smith 2005). The point of IE is to consider the kinds of actions that are prescribed, as well as those foreclosed, in and through specific documentary texts.

A Critical Literature Review

IE distinguishes itself from other kinds of sociological investigation in part because of its commitment to generating useful knowledge. As Marie Campbell and Frances Gregor (2002) argue, thinking about what counts as useful knowledge and conceiving of the 'line of fault' between the knowledge of everyday people and that of the government, requires that scholars remain deeply critical of 'knowledge' itself. One of the ways this is achieved, in practical terms, is in a review of the scholarly literature itself: 'An institutional ethnographer reads the literature, not necessarily for information, but to analyze how the work of intellectuals has helped to give shape to the topic of interest. Institutional ethnographers do not cede authority to the literature, as scholars conventionally do' (7–8). A critical review of the scholarly literature on a topic, then, becomes another instance to understand how and why a particular issue is framed in a specific way. George Smith demonstrates this tactic eloquently in his work on HIV/AIDS. He shows how the public health response to the epidemic, which relies on a clinical definition of AIDS as fatal, forecloses the possibility of thinking about treatment. His review of the available knowledge does not accept it at face value, but rather recognizes research as itself part of the social relation that needs to be understood, explained, and unpacked.

In many ways, our review of epidemiology presented in chapter 1 reflects just such a commitment to maintaining a critical distance from the mainstream scientific scholarship on bisexualities and HIV. We showed the ways in which research on bisexualities reinforces specific racial and cultural stereotypes, underestimates women's vulnerabilities to HIV and other STDs, and in fact erases the realities of bisexual men and women themselves. Our discussion was a critical reading of the research: we think it appropriate, for instance, to question the methodology and design of research that literally makes some research subjects disappear from view! This critical reading also emerges out of a different kind of knowledge that we have of the issues: we know that bisexual men and women exist, even if they cannot prove it in ways acceptable to social scientists. We know that women are at risk of HIV and STD transmission, even if mainstream epidemiology does not bother to ask this question. This knowledge situates us, in the terms of IE, along a line of fault – on the other side of what is 'known' about bisexualities and HIV in official sites of research and policy. The dissonance of such different kinds of knowledge can inform how we approach the 'scientific' literature in this field.

If IE encourages a critical approach to scholarship on a subject, and if it examines how social relations are organized through specific documents, the framework offers a productive model for helping us to think more clearly about how the world is organized, and how knowledge is central to ruling relations. If we wish to consider why there is so little HIV education for men and women with bisexual behaviour in Canada, then, we can use the framework of IE in order to understand more fully how HIV prevention is actually organized and put into place. The following section considers a central policy document in HIV prevention Canada. Analysis of this particular document can help explain how and why certain populations and realities are still without HIV education adapted to their needs more than twenty-five years into an epidemic.

Leading Together: HIV/AIDS Policy in Canada and How It Informs Education

Like most industrialized countries, Canada has produced a number of HIV/AIDS educational initiatives to slow and or stop the transmission of HIV. The importance of such work is significant: HIV is an infectious disease whose consequences are extraordinarily costly for health care systems, and the economy more broadly (CPHA 2005). If there have been a number of different educational campaigns and initiatives – here, the reader may call to mind particular television, newspaper, or billboard advertisements – one still needs to consider how the education that is available is created and distributed. Who makes decisions in this regard, and on what basis? What communities are particularly affected, and how might education be adapted to their particular needs? Who produces such education? Is there a framework that helps answer these questions, that offers a coordinated response to HIV/AIDS education across Canada? If so, what does it say, and why does this matter? We consider these questions throughout this chapter, in order to understand how resources are allocated in the realm of HIV/AIDS prevention.

Close reading of a central policy document in HIV/AIDS can help shed light on these matters. The document in question is entitled *Leading Together: Canada Takes Action on HIV/AIDS (2005–2010)* (CPHA 2005). *Leading Together* is designed to be a strategic document for our response to HIV/AIDS in the current years. It seeks to synthesize research results, identify priorities for action, and make concrete recommendations on how we can act and why. We begin our analysis with a more detailed summary of this document, to familiarize the reader with the appropriate context and background. From there, we engage in a more critical reading of this text in order to show how research informs education. Moreover, we consider the ways in which this document structures our response to HIV/AIDS such that the realities of men and women with bisexual behaviour, as well as their specific vulnerabilities to HIV, are ignored.

Developed through partnership with key stakeholders in the field (community organizations, people living with HIV/AIDS, government policymakers, researchers), *Leading Together* offers a blueprint for action on HIV/AIDS in Canada. It demands critical reflection and action on the issue.

Leading Together challenges governments, organizations, and individuals to:

- make strategic decisions about how to use our resources,
- identify priorities and actions (i.e., some organizations may have a role to play in all aspects of the document, some may be involved in only one activity, and some may select a few priorities that fit within their mandate and resources),
- set out their plans to 2010 and consider how they will contribute to achieving the pan-Canadian targets, desired outcomes, goals, and vision described in the document,
- use the document to build better working relationships with other organizations that serve the same communities or share common goals,
- monitor their initiatives and report on progress, and
- participate in ongoing efforts to ensure the document continues to reflect the optimal response to HIV in Canada, given that the plan will need to evolve as the epidemic and its response continue to shift (CPHA 2005, 3).

Leading Together is central to the federal government's response to the epidemic, and thus linked to the federal initiative on HIV/AIDS.[3] The specific goals outlined in *Leading Together* correspond to the overall objectives of the federal initiative:

1 Reduce the social inequities, stigma, and discrimination that threaten people's health and well-being.
2 Prevent the spread of HIV.
3 Provide timely, safe, and effective diagnosis, care, treatment, and support for all people living in Canada with HIV/AIDS.
4 Contribute to global efforts to fight the epidemic and find a cure (CPHA 2005, 5).

In short, then, this document coordinates the actions of different instances and actors involved in HIV/AIDS in Canada – from the local AIDS Service Organization in Moncton, New Brunswick, to Aboriginal health service providers, to policymakers, to HIV/AIDS researchers in the basic, clinical, epidemiological, and social sciences. Like other strategic planning documents, *Leading Together* provides the framework for people to make sense of and organize their activities.

Having established its objectives, terms of reference, and link to the federal initiative, *Leading Together* goes on to make an argument for the importance of coordinated action in this field. Through a review of the most current scientific literature – particularly clinical, epidemiological, surveillance, and social scientific data – as well as through a consideration of lessons learned from HIV/AIDS since its inception, the document suggests that action is needed for ten reasons:

• The epidemic is increasing.
• People living with HIV/AIDS have increasingly complex needs.
• Too many people with HIV are not receiving – or are resistant to – treatment, and too many are dying.
• Stigma and discrimination continue to threaten people with HIV and communities at risk.
• Poverty, homelessness, and other social determinants are fuelling the epidemic.
• Misconceptions are leading to more risk-taking and less support for services.
• The global epidemic is devastating poorer countries and threatening richer ones.
• Increased and sustainable funding sources are needed to keep pace with the epidemic.

- Acting now will save the health system millions of dollars.
- Acting now will save lives (CPHA 2005, 6–13).

For each of these sections, the document marshals appropriate scientific evidence and rationale. For instance, in the section on stigma and discrimination, *Leading Together* cites a study whose results indicate that nearly 30 per cent of respondents would not be comfortable working in the same office as someone with HIV, while 43 per cent of parents surveyed expressed discomfort at the idea of their child attending school where another child was HIV-positive (CPHA 2005, 9; EKOS Research Associates 2003). In this way, *Leading Together* offers relevant data to inform action. The ten reasons outlined in the document provide a justification of sustained and coordinated action over the five-year period.

This text goes on to outline key principles to be used in actions stemming from the plan (CPHA 2005, 15–17). In the words of the document itself, 'We have identified nine critical success factors or ways of working that, when woven together, form a cohesive blueprint for a coordinated and strategic Canadian response to get ahead of the epidemic (14). These nine key components include:

1 *A commitment to social justice and human rights*. Here, the document underlines the importance of respecting and defending the rights of the vulnerable in society.
2 *Leadership and innovation*. This section outlines the importance of leadership in an effective response to the epidemic. It highlights the significant leadership demonstrated by the gay male community in the fight against HIV/AIDS, particularly in the earlier years of the epidemic.
3 *Meaningful participation of people living with HIV, and communities at risk*. This principle recognizes the importance of involving people with HIV and communities at risk in policy and programming related to HIV. It includes the assertion that 'every effort must be made to encourage meaningful participation, particularly by people and groups who have not been actively involved to date' (PHAC 2005, 16).
4 *Early intervention*. This notion underlines the fact that the best responses to HIV are quick. Countries that implemented needle-exchange programs in the early years of the epidemic, for example, have much lower rates of HIV among injection drug users than nations that did not introduce such services.

5 *Research/evidence.* Here, *Leading Together* champions the role of research in orienting our response to the disease. Research can:
   - enable us to track and monitor the spread of HIV
   - contribute to worldwide efforts to understand and stop HIV disease
   - help us understand the needs of people living with HIV and of communities at risk
   - lead to stronger care and treatment programs
   - inform policy
   - help us make more effective use of limited resources (e.g., financial dependence, violence, abuse, pregnancy and reproduction issues). (CPHA 2005, 17)
6 *A sustained response.* Services and our response to HIV/AIDS cannot be piecemeal or short-sighted solutions. A long-term, sustainable response to the disease is required.
7 *Culture-, gender-, and age-appropriate programs and services.* This principle recognizes that a 'one size fits all' approach to HIV/AIDS prevention and services is inadequate. The importance of tailoring projects to the specific needs of gay men, women, Aboriginal people, and youth is underlined.
8 *A commitment to monitoring, evaluation, and quality improvement.* The document here confirms the importance of monitoring what we do, and learning from experience.
9 *Shared responsibility.* HIV is a complex disease, and its consequences affect many areas of an individual's life. This principle acknowledges that an effective response needs to include different kinds of agencies and actors – for instance, income support programs, correctional services, and housing agencies.

Taken together, these nine 'critical success factors' (CPHA 2005, 14) are to inform our coordinated response to HIV/AIDS.

Leading Together continues with a section outlining shared responsibility, discussing the important role played by different actors. First Nation communities, people living with HIV/AIDS, AIDS service organizations, housing groups, researchers, provincial and federal governments, shelters for battered women, and services for people who use injection drugs are just some of the specific actors named. This section insists on the mutual collaboration of these groups and individuals. HIV/AIDS requires that all of these actors share responsibility in responding to the disease.

All of the previous information presented – objectives of the plan and its link to the federal initiative, justification for action in this area, success factors that must be implemented in all initiatives, and a shared responsibility amongst all actors – provides the necessary background to articulate concrete activities in the field of HIV/AIDS that will have a meaningful impact. In keeping with the principles and approaches outlined above, *Leading Together* proposes six strategies for action:

1 Increase awareness of the impact of HIV/AIDS and increase the commitment to sustained funding for HIV/AIDS programs and services.
2 Address the social factors/inequities driving the epidemic.
3 Step up prevention efforts.
4 Strengthen diagnosis, care, treatment, and support services.
5 Provide leadership in global efforts.
6 Enhance the frontline capacity to act early and stay the course (CPHA 2005, 22).

Taken together, these strategies will have an impact on the different aspects of HIV/AIDS – from prevention to support services to policy – and will help to slow the spread of HIV in Canada, as well as mitigate its consequences.

Each specific strategy is discussed in detail, and for each strategy named, there is an overview of the evidence and rationale specific to it, a naming of desired outcomes, fixed targets to the year 2010,[4] and some proposed actions and recommendations. For example, for the strategy of increasing awareness of HIV/AIDS, the document presents empirical evidence that demonstrates the lack of awareness and misconceptions about HIV. It goes on to then identify the need for increased knowledge of HIV in Canada (desired outcome). Specific targets include the specification that 'by 2010, the proportion of the Canadian public that has misconceptions of HIV/AIDS drops by 50%' (CPHA 2005, 25). Precise actions in this realm include strategic media and communication plans, as well as ensuring that HIV education is a required element of school curricula. This model of rationale, desired outcomes, fixed targets, and actions is applied to each of the six key strategies outlined in *Leading Together* and listed above.

In the next section, we examine the specific strategy named 'Step up prevention efforts' in more depth. Through a consideration of the text's appeal to research, the naming of desired outcomes, the targets fixed, as well as the concrete recommendations and actions proposed, we demonstrate how this document excludes the realities of individuals who have sexual relations with both men and women. Careful analysis of its absences and structural logic can assist us in better understanding how knowledge about HIV/AIDS is produced and taken up in the work of prevention, as well as who gets left out of the picture.

'Step Up Prevention Efforts'

The section of *Leading Together* devoted to HIV/AIDS prevention is one of the six strategies for action named. Given the importance of prevention in controlling the spread of and eradicating HIV in Canada, as well as the costs associated with new HIV diagnoses for the state, this element of *Leading Together* occupies a significant place. The section begins with the statement that 'HIV is first and foremost a preventable disease' and goes on to name specific populations that are at particular risk of HIV infection. Relying on epidemiological surveillance data, *Leading Together*'s reflections on prevention cites several populations in particular: gay men, people who use injection drugs, Aboriginal people, people from countries where HIV is endemic, people in correctional facilities, women and heterosexual transmission, at-risk youth, and babies born to women with HIV. For each of these populations, the document outlines targets and actions as part of its prevention response to HIV. Close analysis of this text helps to explain the virtual absence of bisexual men and women as a population within Canadian AIDS policy.

The neglect of bisexual men and women in prevention is amply evidenced in the section entitled 'Gay Men.' While the section title is that of 'gay men,' the document is quick to also invoke the realities of bisexual men, at least in theory. Indeed, this part of the document opens with the rationale for the impact of HIV among gay and bisexual men: 'MSM (including gay and bisexual men) continue to be the group most affected by HIV/AIDS. In 2002, they accounted for 58% of the 56,000 people living with HIV infection and 40% of all new infections (an increase from 38% of new infections in 1999). Over the last few years, there has also been an increase in the number of MSM diagnosed with other STIs, such as syphilis. These trends indicate that gay men are engaging in riskier sexual behaviours' (CPHA 2005, 30). The introduction to reflection on prevention among MSM, then, names bisexual men specifically. Yet only two sentences later, bisexual men have been disregarded: the document does not tell us if there is an indication of trends of riskier behaviour among bisexual men. Rather, it extrapolates from MSM data to make statements about the sexual practices of gay men.

Such complex and contradictory relations between the categories 'gay men,' 'bisexual men,' and 'MSM' are omnipresent within this section of the document. In a discussion of one particular educational campaign, the document includes an inset box with the heading 'How Do You Know What You Know? A Prevention Campaign Targeting Gay Men' (CPHA 2005, 31). However, within the description of this initiative, in smaller type, the document proclaims that organizations across the country 'are participating in a prevention campaign that targets gay and bisexual men' (31). It then quickly states that the 'campaign challenges gay men to review the strategies they use to assess risk and to challenge the assumptions they make about their sexual partners' (31). Once again, bisexual men seem to appear – in the fine print – only to disappear from view. Prevention initiatives that rely on MSM data and include bisexual men actually provide little reflection on the specific needs of bisexual men. In the Assumptions campaign discussed above, for example, the images are those of anal sex between men. Sex with a woman (whether vaginal or anal), and assumptions about a male bisexual's female partners, have not been addressed. In this regard, the educational campaign has been created for gay men in particular – a discourse of 'MSM' or 'gay and bisexual men' notwithstanding. This example helps to understand the specific lack of attention to bisexual men's lives. Indeed, rhetorical appeals to 'MSM' or 'gay and bisexual men' give the impression that this reality has been addressed – bisexual men are at least named within this policy document (which is more than can be said for bisexual women). Yet the educational initiatives that stem from such policy orientations are actually rather ignorant of bisexual men's lives, since they somehow imagine that it is acceptable to develop educational materials for bisexual men that neglect their female partners entirely.

Research is fundamental to the framing of this policy document, and thus to the exclusion of bisexuality. In its reflections on prevention among MSM and gay men, *Leading Together* invokes two recent studies of challenges and factors to take into consideration, including the assumptions gay men make about their (male) partners, as well as the fact that many are knowledgeable about HIV/AIDS. Specific issues that are particular to bisexual men, however, are absent from the discussion – even though the studies on which these policy orientations are based invoked (at least in principle) 'gay and bisexual men' (CPHA 2005, 30). Such relations between research and knowledge are made explicit in *Leading Together*: 'These research findings are being used to develop prevention strategies that engage the gay community in discussions on how to interpret risk messages, negotiate safety and manage relationships' (31). Here again, there is an implicit and exclusive reference to gay male communities. In this way, *Leading Together* consolidates the erasure of bisexuals within a broader MSM category, since there is a sustained refusal to consider any data from MSM research that might be specific to bisexual men and women.

While the exclusion of bisexuality within discourse is most notable in the section of the document related to MSM and gay men, it can also be observed elsewhere in the reflections on prevention. Within a specific attention to at-risk youth, for example, *Leading Together* states that certain youth are increasingly vulnerable to HIV infection, among them those who use injection drugs, gay youth, and Aboriginal youth. While such a statement is not to be discounted, it is noteworthy that only gay youth are mentioned as sexual minorities. Indeed, consideration of empirical research in the field indicates that bisexual men and women experience more social isolation and suicidal feelings than either heterosexuals or lesbians and gay men (ISQ 1998). Furthermore, bisexuals are subject to more violence than either lesbians and gays or heterosexuals – while lesbians and gay men experience rates of violence 2.5 times those of heterosexual men and women, bisexuals experience 4 times the rate of violent incidents against heterosexuals (Statistics Canada 2008). Given the attention that *Leading Together* gives to the social factors that increase vulnerability to HIV (CPHA 2005, 11), an absence of attention to the specific situation of bisexual youth is conspicuous.

One final example of the problematic citation of bisexuality within *Leading Together* appears in the section on prevention specific to women, 'Women and Heterosexual Transmission.' Bisexual men do appear in this section but are cited in particular as a potential risk factor for heterosexual women. The section opens with a review of the rise in new HIV infections amongst women in Canada (over a quarter of new infections in 2004), and claims, 'Many of the women are Aboriginal, from a country where HIV is endemic, users of injection drugs or are at risk from sex with a partner who injects drugs or who has had sex with men' (CPHA 2005, 35). Here, bisexual men are presented as a risk factor – note that the text does not refer to men who have had *unprotected* sexual relations with other men. The issue is not that a woman has sex with a man who has had sexual relations with another man.

HIV can be transmitted through sexual intercourse only when the sexual relation between the woman and the man is unprotected, as well as when the sexual relation between the two men was unprotected. Yet this document does not make such a careful distinction (which is instructive, more than twenty-five years into an epidemic). Rather, surveillance data are used to speak about 'risk groups' – those who use injection drugs, Aboriginal people, and bisexual men. In this regard, the discussion of heterosexual transmission of HIV imagines that sex with a bisexual man is a factor in itself for HIV transmission – a position that ignores the basic science of how the virus is transmitted and continues to focus on questions of *who* people are as opposed to *what* they do. Indeed, HIV/AIDS activists have long challenged this narrow way of thinking about HIV and have demanded that education speak about what people do, not who they are (Patton 2002; Shephard Heim 1997). While there has certainly been some success in this regard with gay men in particular (Patton), it appears that the scenario is somewhat different for bisexual men. This framing of bisexual men as potential vectors of infection, present within a national policy document published in 2005, indicates the extent to which cultural stereotypes about the diseased and duplicitous bisexual man persist (Miller 2002). This scapegoating of bisexual men in particular stands in ironic relation to the reflections on stigma and discrimination presented in the broader document (CPHA 2005, 26–9).

The section of *Leading Together* that devotes itself to prevention, then, configures bisexuality in very specific ways. On the one hand, in certain instances, bisexual men are targeted as vectors of infection, those who transmit HIV to heterosexual women. Despite blaming them for the transmission of HIV, however, the document actually provides very little – if any – reflection on the specific challenges involved in developing HIV prevention for men who have sexual relations with both men and women. Although bisexuals are mentioned within a broader discussion of MSM, such an invocation is rhetorical at best. *Leading Together* provides no sustained reflection on data relevant to bisexual lives, and the targets, outcomes, and actions it names within the field of MSM are specific to gay men.

It is important to examine how this document neglects relevant information on the lives of bisexuals entirely: the ways in which only certain kinds of knowledge and research are invoked and discussed. But from the perspective of institutional ethnography, one must also consider what this text does. *Leading Together* is a strategic planning document. It is designed to provide an overview of the current situation, and to set out ambitious targets, outcomes, and actions in order to respond more adequately to the challenges of HIV. *Leading Together*, then, seeks to provide a frame of reference for the everyday work that is to be done – from HIV prevention, to community education, to research. In this manner, the document is central to understanding and organizing the response to HIV in Canada. It does more than simply offer a commentary on the situation. It outlines the actions required so that we respond collectively to HIV/AIDS in all its complexity. Like other strategic planning documents, *Leading Together* organizes the daily administrative work. It is, in the language of Dorothy Smith (2006, 86), a 'regulatory text.' A regulatory text determines the scope and frame of action in a specific area. It subordinates other texts to its logic. For example, as a regulatory text, *Leading Together* provides the framework to make sense of future initiatives within HIV/AIDS in Canada. It is a policy document that is used to make sense of and create other kinds of texts, such as HIV/AIDS educational materials and campaigns. Because of this central administrative role, absences within *Leading Together* will persist. Since it has not considered relevant data on bisexual men and women, and since it does not name any actions specific to HIV education with bisexual men and women, the text also perpetuates the exclusion of bisexuals from research, policy, and education. *Leading Together* works as a regulatory text to coordinate and organize other work in HIV/AIDS, providing the framework to be taken up. Since bisexual men and women have been made invisible therein, it is not surprising to remark the absence of HIV prevention specific to bisexuality in general within Canada.

In order to understand more clearly why there is a dearth of HIV education for bisexual men and women in Canada, it is instructive to consider certain kinds of central policy documents. Our discussion here has examined the ways in which *Leading Together*, a national strategic planning document on HIV/AIDS action, repeats stereotypes about bisexual men and literally erases bisexual men and women from consideration in HIV/AIDS prevention. The centrality of such a policy for future action on HIV/AIDS helps to explain how and why the specific needs of bisexual men and women continue to be overlooked.

In the next section, we expand our analysis in this regard, through a consideration of HIV/AIDS funding and its institutional organization. Reflection on some of the invisible ways in which HIV/AIDS funding is organized will provide further insight into the exclusion of bisexual men and women from prevention education in Canada.

Funding HIV/AIDS Research in Canada

To state that this research project confronted difficulties in securing funding would be an understatement. While the project obtained a grant from the Social Sciences and Humanities Research Council of Canada (SSHRC) in 2004, it is noteworthy that many different versions of this particular grant were presented to different funding bodies. We recount some of our experience in the granting process here. The point is not to complain or lament the review process. Rather, by attending to the justification of a grant being refused, or funded, we can better understand how the institutions responsible for research funding operate – what they take for granted, the kinds of knowledge they value, and the level of scientific rigour required in applications. Until now we have considered some of the profound limitations of research on bisexualities and HIV/AIDS. This knowledge will be supplemented with an in-depth appreciation of how decisions about HIV/AIDS research funding get made, and what kinds of projects may be lost within such institutional workings. As we will soon see, it is necessary to comprehend how and why research on HIV/AIDS is framed in order to appreciate why there has been no critical research on bisexualities and HIV/AIDS in Canada.

'More Information about the Prevalence of Bisexuality within the Studied Population'

We begin with an anecdote taken from a grant submitted to SSHRC in 2002. The committee was relatively favourable to our proposal, but did express some reservations. In particular, committee members wished to have 'more information about the prevalence of bisexuality within the studied population.'[5] Before we unpack this statement, a few words on the operations of peer review committees are in order. Academic research funded by bodies like SSHRC demands a process known as 'peer review.' This means that one's colleagues have reviewed all proposals for funding. Applications are sent first to two reviewers, who prepare reports to be considered at a larger committee meeting. This larger committee then examines all applications, including the external reports, and makes recommendations on which projects should be funded. This is an extraordinarily difficult job, and hard choices must be made: applications are ranked in order of funding priority, with the keen knowledge that there will be a specific cut-off point after which applications are not likely to be funded. Because of the volume of applications, as well as supporting materials, committees prepare summary reports on the strengths and weaknesses of each grant application. They summarize the committee discussion and communicate it to applicants so that they can improve their proposal for a future round of funding. The comment on our grant application cited above came from this committee summary.

Yet let us consider the comment in more depth, for it is revealing. The grant review committee wished to have more information about the occurrence of bisexuality within a sample population of bisexuals. The logic here is of the same order of that discussed within general public health research on HIV/AIDS. (The committee in question included health sciences in its mandate.) The reviewers wanted to know, in effect, about the sexual practices of bisexual men and women – the 'prevalence' of bisexuality itself. This comment adheres to a specific understanding of bisexuality in which bisexuality is, as we have seen, fleeting and unstable – hence the need to provide more descriptive data of the referent in question. We do not feel, for instance, that a grant committee would write to an applicant, 'We would like to have more information about the prevalence of homosexuality in a population of gay men,' or that they would demand precision on the 'prevalence of heterosexuality within a study on teenage sexual mores.' The comment tells us, then, about the difficulties in imagining bisexuality itself. Furthermore, the invocation of a notion of 'prevalence' is firmly situated within a specific logic of behaviour-based inquiry. This framework is less relevant for our research, since we are concerned about people's HIV information needs. Moreover, the comment does seem to belie a fundamental contradiction: our review of the scientific literature in the field noted the dearth of studies on bisexualities, particularly in Canada. At the time we submitted the application, there had been no large-scale empirical study of bisexual men and women in Canada. Yet committee members responded with the request for more information about the sample population's characteristics – as if such data could simply be cited. Indeed, funding this proposal would provide some empirical data in the Canadian context. Our proposal was caught in a circular logic – empirical studies on bisexualities could not be funded because, well, we don't have enough background information about the empirical realities of bisexuals in order to evaluate the proposal.

Having received this feedback, we resubmitted the proposal. There, we outlined the difficulties raised by this comment – the way in which it imposed criteria of empiricism that would not, in our view, be applied to other sexualities, and the manner in which the comment itself demonstrates the profound epistemological difficulties in thinking about bisexuals. Fortunately, committee members received our critical response favourably and funded the application in 2004.

Our experience with this committee is instructive, however. It demonstrates the profound difficulty in doing innovative research that breaks with previous academic scholarship. Moreover, within the field of sexuality studies, our experience shows the ways in which misconceptions about sexuality can be operationalized institutionally: the confusion over bisexuality in and of itself was a central justification in arguing that our proposal should not be funded. Of course, our experience is not necessarily unique, perhaps especially in the field of HIV/AIDS. In an insightful analysis of the review process of HIV/AIDS research in the United States, Peter Gould (1993) recounts the profound difficulties that he experienced in obtaining funding for his work on the geography of AIDS. Briefly, Gould is a geographer interested in considering the spatial dimensions of disease. He began to think about the spread of HIV not just through time – the number of new infections in a given year – but also through space, tracking the ways new infections could literally be mapped, following the routes of travellers and citizens on the move. Gould's work sought to track these spatial developments – to map the way HIV in the United States had New York City as one of its first epicentres, but also how it quickly fanned out beyond this metropolis to other urban centres, and eventually to more rural regions over time. Moreover, he wanted to think through the predictive value of such spatial thinking. If one can track the way HIV moves across geographic boundaries, locating the cities, towns, and counties where it gains entry and multiplies, then one can also use these data to make decisions about where to allocate prevention resources. If you know, for example, that HIV is moving from Cleveland to Cincinnati to more rural counties in Ohio, you can engage in some innovative prevention education before the numbers of HIV rise dramatically in Cincinnati. While Gould was committed to developing this kind of geographic analysis of HIV and of linking its relevance to prevention, he had difficulty in having the validity of his perspective recognized within the established AIDS research infrastructure, dominated by clinical scientists and epidemiologists. Gould's work was in some ways at odds with traditional epidemiology and public health, which examines disease temporally (for instance, the notion of incidence, the number of new infections in a given year). He sought to consider disease spatially and temporally and to test some educational tools that incorporated these conceptions of HIV/AIDS in order to do prevention work. He implicitly questioned the traditional epidemiological framework for doing research and comments on the difficulties encountered:

> But the review panel of NIH (National Institutes of Health), loaded with MDs, conventional epidemiologists, and a 'senior behavioral scientist' (his actual title), had never heard of the national call for interdisciplinary research, and they were distinctly unsympathetic to anything so useful as producing materials for educational intervention. You have to understand the close-knit nature of many reviewing panels, most of them formed from a relatively small pool of Establishment team players. Blinkered by the paradigms they were taught at graduate school years before, it is quite clear to them that there are only a few ways in which a scientific task can be approached. Most of them publish in esoteric journals of limited circulation, and would not dream of doing anything that could be constrained as practical with their research. (Gould 1993, 148)

This extract reveals the ways in which decisions about funding are far from neutral. They reflect the specific interests and expertise of committee members and often reinforce existing paradigms of knowledge. For researchers who are thinking outside the established box, this can present a serious challenge. The experience of Gould, as well as our own experience with SSHRC cited above, is instructive in a critical analysis of funding HIV/AIDS research. These anecdotes raise important questions: What kinds of paradigms are the norm within HIV/AIDS research? What research is there on sexual minorities in general, and on bisexuals in particular? What are some of the additional burdens of proof required of applicants whose work does not follow traditional frameworks of knowledge? What types of HIV/AIDS research projects get funded overall? What kinds of research projects are refused funding, and with what justification? What are the ways in which some of the gaps in HIV/AIDS research are directly related to the ways that research funding is organized?

Whose Community?

An experience with a different funding body reveals related difficulties in securing the monies required to do this empirical research. The specific fund in question, Community-Based HIV/AIDS Research Programme, is housed at the Canadian Institutes of Health Research (CIHR). A bit of history of this funding program is in order. The idea behind it is to create an opportunity for communities to conduct research that addresses the epidemic. In the late 1990s, some AIDS organizers in Montréal made the compelling argument to government that while there was a great deal of research on HIV/AIDS, affected and infected communities were not always involved. The practice of community-based research (CBR) was advocated. CBR advances a number of key principles, including relevance (that the research conducted be pertinent to the people at hand), initiative (that the research emerge from the community), ownership (that the community own the knowledge generated), and equity (that all partners – academic, community, public health – have an equal say and equal participation). CBR is an effort to have everyday people involved in producing knowledge about their lives. Within the field of HIV/AIDS, it is promoted as especially relevant, so that research does not simply identify academic priorities but serves the people under investigation. In the late 1990s, Québec AIDS organizers promoted this model of research and argued that community organizations needed to develop their capacity to conduct research. They lobbied the federal government for funds in this area and obtained a research facilitator. This person, knowledgeable about HIV/AIDS, community organizations, and research funding, would work with local community organizations to develop research questions they deemed relevant, and eventually to submit applications for funding. The program was important to legitimize the knowledge within community-based HIV/AIDS organizations, to help foster a culture of reflection and research within such sites, and to facilitate access to research monies. This last point was especially important for community organizations, who traditionally had no access to research funding because they were unable to obtain ethical approval for their research. The program has been housed in a number of different institutional sites, beginning with the National Health Research and Development Programme, then Health Canada, and finally the Canadian Institutes of Health Research, where it currently resides. Although it began in Québec, this program has expanded across Canada – research technical associates are funded in several regions across Canada, and the program funds operating grants, seed grants, and capacity-development workshops. There is a similar program specific to Aboriginal people and HIV/AIDS in Canada, ensuring that Aboriginal people are equal partners in the knowledge generated about their lives.

In 2002, we prepared a grant application to seek funding for this project, presented to Health Canada, the administrative body then responsible for administering the Community-Based HIV/AIDS Research Programme. We were particularly enthusiastic about this fund: here was a funding program that recognized the importance of involving people and communities who had historically been excluded from knowledge itself. Given the neglect of bisexuality within HIV/AIDS research, we were optimistic about our proposal, since it brought together bisexual organizers and activists in Montréal to conduct some CBR on the HIV prevention needs of bisexual men and women.

Our application included letters of support from local bisexual organizations, Bi Unité Montréal and Bi Montréal, as well as a number of local bisexuals who expressed support for the project. Moreover, the organizers of 'Soirées polyvalence' were involved (Vukov, Williamson, Namaste), since this experience in organizing social parties for bisexuals represented sound knowledge of bisexual communities and networks in Montréal. We proposed, as well, a community-based advisory committee to oversee the project, with representatives from the organizations and people above. In all of these ways, this project was a community endeavour. Indeed, this initiative was to our knowledge the first instance in Canada of bisexual men and women coming together to identify our own research question and to propose a large-scale empirical study.

The evaluating committee did not rate the application favourably enough to obtain funding. In its justification, the committee stated that the project was not 'community-based' and specified that a letter of support from a provincial network of gay and bisexual HIV/AIDS organizations was not included with the application as a demonstration of community support.[6] This comment, and the specific appeal to such a provincial network of HIV/AIDS groups, is revealing. The reference here is to la Coalition des organismes communautaires dans la lutte contre le SIDA (COCQ-Sida), a provincial network of HIV/AIDS agencies. (That said, the COCQ-Sida does not have any bisexual associations among its members, which leads us to the conclusion that the committee's comments reflect an ignorance of the Québec AIDS milieu: there is no provincial coalition of gay and bisexual HIV/AIDS groups.) Perhaps more significantly, the comment suggests that 'community' is to be defined within the terms of HIV/AIDS groups already recognized and funded by the state. Our project was not judged to be 'community-based,' since we had not provided the appropriate documentation from such groups in the application. But curiously, the documentation that we had provided from bisexual organizations, activists, social party organizers, and interested individuals was simply overlooked. Within this discourse, bisexuals cannot write a letter and be 'community.' Bisexuals cannot represent themselves; they need the authorization of provincial AIDS groups – a curious argument within the terms of a grant application that is supposed to be about communities organizing to identify their own needs and to do their own research. This line of argument, in our view, follows that articulated by our SSHRC evaluation: no one can imagine who these bisexuals actually are. (We're seeing a definite pattern here in research on bisexualities!)

Furthermore, the criterion that we submit a letter from the COCQ-Sida in order to demonstrate our community base follows a somewhat perverse logic. Our research proposal illustrates the ways in which there is virtually no research or education on bisexualities and HIV/AIDS in Canada. In this light, HIV/AIDS agencies have shown no particular expertise on this population. More critically, such agencies are in some ways part of the problem, to the extent that they avoid sustained reflection and action on a population blamed for the transmission of HIV (bisexual men in particular). To require a letter of support from established HIV/AIDS agencies as proof of community relevance is to demand that a particular initiative secure the backing and endorsement of the very agencies who have neglected bisexual populations. Within such a logic, the exclusion of populations like bisexuals from an established HIV/AIDS infrastructure cannot be addressed, since these organizations hold the sole proprietary right to be 'community' under the terms of the program (at least as interpreted by this particular evaluation committee). This comment, then, helps us to understand who counts as 'community' within AIDS funding, as well as some of the reasons why there is so little research conducted that is highly critical, or simply not within the usual boundaries, of established HIV/AIDS groups. Moreover, this situation suggests that there is a lack of critical reflection on the limits of 'community-based research' as a concept and a practice in itself (Mykalovskiy and Cain 2008).

The refusal of our grant application on the grounds that the proposal was not 'community-based' reflects more than the opinions of one peer evaluation committee. This situation illustrates some of the profound transformations of community organizations that have occurred within the past three decades, as well as current understandings of the role and function of community agencies. Eric Shragge's (2003) work on local and community organizing can assist us here. Shragge, a long-time community organizer and academic, reflects on the manner in which community organizations have transformed since the 1960s in Québec. He traces the development of these agencies rooted in responding to everyday people's problems. A strong ethic of solidarity and user participation was prominent in such organizations in the early days; Shragge cites the examples of community health clinics (initiated in the 1960s when health care was still privatized in Québec) that had neighbourhood and community residents on the clinic's board of directors. These kinds of initiatives offered services, but they also engaged in popular education and grassroots mobilization. With the advent of neoliberalism beginning in the 1980s, however, the definition of the role of a community organization changed dramatically. The retreat and withdrawal of the welfare state meant that programs and services previously offered by public institutions were downloaded to community organizations – at a fraction of the cost. This created a different context in which community organizations entered more frequently into contractual and funding arrangements with the state. Importantly, such agencies increasingly turned their mandate to service provision, developing funding proposals to fulfil specific needs. On the one hand, of course, this is a positive development insofar as the state recognizes the innovative and important contributions of community organizations. On the other hand, it is significant that such recognition does not come with allocation of resources parallel to those previously allocated to the public sector. Moreover, such a context reshapes the daily work of organizations in which service provision takes precedence. Shragge argues that this trend was only reinforced in the 1990s, such that matters of popular education and grassroots mobilization were put on the back-burner for most state-funded agencies: 'Community organizations were faced with the dilemma that greater recognition and funding actually diminished their autonomy and reinforced a service agenda. With this orientation, groups shifted from a membership or social movement base to a client focus. This redefinition is inherently depoliticizing. Clients are to be served and have a less active – or no – role in either the organizations' internal processes or on wider social issues. At best, they are represented rather than mobilized. Thus, the form of political representation became lobbying by coalitions of community organizations promoting the needs of a particular population' (Shragge 2003, 55).

The complicated relations between community organizations and the state outlined by Shragge are examined with specific reference to HIV/AIDS by Gary Kinsman (1992). Kinsman considers key policy documents in the management of HIV/AIDS at the end of the 1980s, an era marked by neoliberalism and the retreat of the state in the provision of health care and social services. His analysis considers the manner in which the government appealed to 'partnership' between federal funding agencies and community organizations. Acknowledging the recognition of community groups that this afforded – a key idea advanced by activists since the inception of the AIDS epidemic – Kinsman also underlines the fact that this idea of 'partnership' transformed agencies into service providers – leaving matters of grassroots mobilization to the side. Moreover, whereas community groups in the early days of the epidemic were instrumental in naming priorities for political action, a partnership model in which the state funds community groups can also mean that the state is directly involved in the daily work of such organizations: 'A crucial aspect of this partnership strategy is to get other groups, including community groups, to do work for state agencies. This can be seen as subcontracting state work to "community-based" groups through specific funding projects, project guidelines and the work of funding officers. State agencies thus come to shape the deployment of resources and to reshape agendas of community-based groups' (223).

Kinsman provides the details about HIV/AIDS in the scenario outlined by Shragge: a literal transformation of community organizations from sites of popular education and grassroots mobilization to agencies of service provision to clients. As scholars in the field of state policy and the community sector have demonstrated, these social relations were introduced in the late 1970s and early 1980s and were strengthened and intensified throughout the 1990s (Jette 2008; Lamoureux 2007; Orsini 2006; White 1992). The specific incarnation of state–community relations in the 1990s brought such organizations into formal partnership agreements, contracting them to provide services. The introduction of such partnerships in turn reduced genuine citizen involvement significantly (Ravet 2009). Indeed, Shragge discusses the ways in which this shift to a client model transformed the kinds of political action enacted. Within a context of service-provider, client-centred agencies, one can observe political action that is carried out not by everyday people themselves (now reduced to mere clients or users). Rather, larger bodies and coalitions speak for such constituencies. Henri Lamoureux underlines this expert status that community organizations body seek and embody:

> Le citoyen a de moins en moins d'importance aux yeux d'un organisme voué à la prestation de services, qui se considérera par ailleurs comme une entreprise à finalité sociale. Il n'aura guère plus de pouvoir dans un groupe qui se définit comme expert dans un domaine donné et qui cherche à s'imposer comme seul interlocuteur représentatif d'une « clientèle » ciblée, présentant des caractéristiques particulières : les locataires, les femmes, les jeunes, les retraités, les toxicomanes, les prestataires de l'aide social, les personnes handicapées intellectuelles, les « ex-psychiatrisés », etc. (Lamoureux 2007, 52–3)

> (The citizen has less and less importance in the eyes of an organization devoted to providing services, which will therein define itself as a social business. She will hardly have more power in a group that defines itself as an expert within a given field and seeks to impose itself as the sole spokesperson representative of a specific 'clientele' with particular characteristics: tenants, welfare recipients, the intellectually disabled, psychiatric survivors, etc.)[7]

Like Shragge and Kinsman, Lamoureux here draws our attention to the ways in which the very definition and understanding of community organizations has been transformed over the past few decades, and how this transformation is a clear move away from democratic governance of community agencies. This point is echoed by Frédérique Le Goff, Christopher McAll, and Catherine Montgomery, who argue that currently 'ce ne sont que les intervenants maintenant qui siègent aux comités et tables locaux et régionaux pour faire connaître leurs revendications' (now, it is only front-line workers who sit on committees and local and regional boards to voice their concerns) (2005, 162; translation ours).

Theoretically, scholarly writing in this area makes three important points. First, the actual workings of the state have a direct impact on how community organizations are structured (Orsini 2006), perhaps especially within the context of partnership agreements. Second, the community sector is held up as the appropriate 'solution' for the gap in services provided by the state (White 1992), a particular rhetorical move that equates a vague notion of 'community' with ensuring social

and economic justice (Panet Raymond 1994). And finally, current artic-
ulations of relations between community organizations and the state,
in which agencies offer services to clients, involves an implicit model
of community organizations and community organizing – a function-
alist vision of the role of these agencies (organizations enact a specific function clearly delineated by the state: they provide services),
as opposed to a conception of them that includes action in their role
(theoretically, the latter model is situated within the terms of conflict
theory) (Shragge 2005, 70).

These reflections on the role of community organizations are instructive for our consideration of AIDS research funding, and in particular for
evaluating the comment that our proposal was not community-based
because it did not have a letter of support from a provincial network of
HIV/AIDS agencies. This justification displays more than a mere lack
of consideration for bisexual men and women and a disregard for the
letters of support presented by such individuals, activists, and associations. More strongly, the rationale provided for not funding the proposal
appeals to the ultimate force and validity of the provincial network of
HIV/AIDS organizations. Such a comment is possible only in a broader
context in which provincial coalitions of HIV/AIDS actors are seen
to hold truth, expertise, and the right to act. The comment belies the
dynamics of community organizations and the state deftly analysed by
Shragge, Kinsman, and Lamoureux. Everyday people and even associations (bisexuals) cannot guarantee appropriate community input; such
an assurance can be secured only through the involvement of coalitions.
Aside from the fact that no group within such a coalition has produced
educational materials specific to HIV/AIDS and bisexualities in Québec, the mere presence of such a coalition is strong enough to demonstrate 'community.' The evaluation comment sent to us, then, tells us
about the particular understanding of 'community' among committee
members, one limited to agencies already recognized and funded by the
state. Indeed, this particular comment serves as a point of entry for us to
reflect on the particular understanding of the relations between community organizations and the state within the field of HIV/AIDS. The comment appeals to the expert status of certain recognized actors, taking
for granted a model of community in which state-funded services offer
the appropriate response to a particular issue (in this case, HIV/AIDS),
and in which their primary function is to offer services. However, the
exclusion of the bisexual individuals and organizations as 'community'
does more than value certain players and forms of knowledge in the

field. Such a move in fact pre-empts the community organizing and collective action of some people who have sexual relations with both men and women in the field. Paradoxically, the workings of a community-based HIV/AIDS research fund, functioning within the terms of neoliberal state–community relations, prevents initiatives situated outside the terms of a service-provision model, thus reinforcing particularly narrow understandings of 'community.'

We would like to raise two final issues on this experience in our grant submission. In the first instance, the position that one must have coalitions of HIV/AIDS agencies on board in order to obtain funding may, in fact, be counterproductive to conducting innovative research in the field. As we will see when we present the results of our study in more depth, many of the people we interviewed are deeply suspicious of existing HIV/AIDS groups and are highly critical of the prevention education they have seen. Research that is done only with existing groups might not reach people who choose not to access their services, generating partial knowledge and in effect creating an epistemological tautology. Second, this situation illustrates the perverse logic that Kinsman describes, of 'partnership' and inclusion of community groups. The research fund to which this application was submitted – the Community-Based HIV/AIDS Research Progamme of Health Canada – includes parity of academic and community researchers. Academics and community members come together in equal numbers to evaluate all proposals. This is, of course, a hard-won battle: there are few other committees where community members have the same status and say as health scientists in the funding of research. As such, the composition and existence of this committee is an important victory for community activists, and it is crucial to ensure that relevant research be carried out. Conversely, the very composition of the community is also a potential weakness: 'community' is defined through both implicit and explicit reference to state-funded community groups. As our experience in seeking funding has shown, not just any community group or collection of concerned individuals suffices to stand in for 'community.' Indeed, only the most recognized groups are understood to be 'community' in this site. Our experience shows how this particular, limited understanding of 'community' excludes entire populations of people – ironically, populations that have not yet been served by current groups. If the entry of community members into this peer review committee is to be celebrated, it is also to be criticized to the extent that it consolidates the power and status of certain groups as experts, to the exclusion of others.

Our experience in seeking funding for this research has been instructive on a number of levels. The evaluative feedback presented to us is telling, showing, for instance, the ways in which common misconceptions about bisexuals (i.e., do they even exist?) are central to the argument used in evaluating our proposal. Moreover, our dealings with a specifically community-based research fund included the somewhat startling statement that our work was not 'community-based.' Here, a particular definition of 'community' is at play, one overdetermined by the relations between state funding and community organizations within a context of neoliberalism. Our intent in relating these efforts to secure funding is not simply to complain or lament the fact that we did not receive funding. Rather, we seek to unpack the rationale provided in different instances. In this manner, our work is an effort to help clarify the invisible workings of institutions in research funding. We have demonstrated, for instance, the ways in which state-funded community organizations hold a privileged place within an institutional site of community-based research. More critically, our work shows how some representatives of these organizations exclude different populations and communities through an appeal to community expertise of 'recognized' coalitions and groups.

This section on research funding is important, because, in the field of HIV/AIDS, research plays a central role in determining policy, providing justification for funding, orienting action, developing services, and creating education. If we wish to understand why there is no HIV/AIDS education for bisexuals in Canada, we need to examine how decisions about funding HIV/AIDS research are made and the ways such decisions favour existing populations and communities. In the final section of this chapter, we examine the terms and conditions of funding that is available for community-based HIV programming in Canada, through a specific case study. Analysis of one specific grant competition illustrates the ways in which the issues outlined above define the terms and reference of funding mechanisms, and how people and populations like bisexuals are excluded.

Specific Populations: The Exclusion of Bisexuality in Federal AIDS Funding

In this section, we offer a case study of one fund offered as part of the federal initiative on HIV/AIDS: the Specific Populations HIV/AIDS Initiative Fund (which we will refer to as the Specific Populations Fund for the sake of brevity). This fund was created to support national initiatives to prevent the spread of HIV in populations most affected by HIV/AIDS in Canada, as listed in alphabetical order:

- Aboriginal peoples
- Gay men
- People from countries where HIV is endemic
- People living with HIV/AIDS
- People who use injection drugs
- Inmates
- Women at risk
- Youth at risk

Of course, this list is similar to the list of communities identified as relevant in the *Leading Together* document discussed earlier. Indeed, one can see the influence of *Leading Together* in this fund: the populations identified as relevant within the strategic planning document are named within this funding envelope. As a regulatory text, *Leading Together* determines the frame of reference for future policy and programming in the field of HIV/AIDS. It helps name the communities considered 'relevant' for the Specific Populations Fund – the communities considered most affected by HIV/AIDS.

The Specific Populations Fund acknowledges this debt explicitly to *Leading Together* and provides an overview of how priorities were determined for this fund: 'The Populations Fund will have population-specific policy, program and social marketing priorities identified by PHAC through its ongoing assessment of data related to the HIV/AIDS epidemic in Canada, stakeholder consultation and the federal role in supporting the activities, outputs and vision of *Leading Together*. Note that the priorities of subsequent requests for proposals will be modified based on the review of available data' (Specific Populations HIV/AIDS Initiative Fund (2006), Guide for Applicants, p. 4). Elsewhere, the same document describes the process for naming the priorities in more detail: 'Based upon the PHAC[Public Health Agency of Canada]'s review of available epidemiological, statistical and consultative data (such as *Leading Together*), population-specific funding priorities have been established for the 2006 request for proposals for the Populations Fund' (Specific Populations HIV/AIDS Initiative Fund (2006), Guide for Applicants, p. 10).

Having offered an overview of the process to determine priorities, the Specific Populations Fund does allow for nuance in its understanding of populations. The fund welcomes initiatives that strengthen capacity of health-care providers working in HIV/AIDS prevention and names the specific populations listed above. It goes further to also encourage proposals dealing with 'cross-cutting populations' such as

- young gay men, Two Spirit men, men just coming out, older gay men, immigrant men who have sex with men (MSM), and male sex workers,
- Aboriginal people who use injection drugs,
- women who use injection drugs,
- Aboriginal women, and
- female sex workers (Specific Populations HIV/AIDS Initiative Fund (2006), Guide for Applicants, p. 11).

The notion of a 'cross-cutting population' is an effort to acknowledge that people's lives are complicated and often more complex than one identity category deemed relevant within public health. In this regard, this concept is an attempt to avoid the problems of putting people in boxes, as described in our review of epidemiological approaches to disease in chapter 1. Goodwill notwithstanding, we find it significant that bisexual men and women still receive no mention within this idea of 'cross-cutting populations': the further detail given on MSM ignores bisexual men entirely, while bisexual women are also eclipsed.

The arguments we outlined previously help explain how and why bisexuals are not named as priorities within this fund. From the perspective of a review of the available literature, we have argued that much of the most relevant scientific literature on bisexual men and women has been ignored in the *Leading Together* policy document. There is no citation of the poor access bisexuals have to health care services, or of their increased isolation and lack of support – in all instances, empirical data suggest that the situation faced by bisexual men and women is in fact much worse than that faced by lesbians and gay men. Although there is citation of certain MSM studies, there is little or no consideration of data specifically relevant to bisexual men. Nor is there, in our view, a thorough review of the epidemiological literature. In chapter 1, we offered an overview of the epidemiological literature on bisexual women and HIV/STDs, showing through appeal to scientific evidence that bisexual women are more vulnerable to HIV and STDs than either heterosexual women or lesbians. Yet in the Specific Population Funds invocation of 'women at risk,' there is no mention of bisexual women.

They are similarly absent from the *Leading Together* document. Thus, while policy documents and the fund application guide contend that the priorities named are based on a review of the scientific literature, our research shows that the survey of the data has not considered women's sexual lives in their diversity. The irony of this situation – to fail to conduct a complete literature review of sexuality and sexual orientations when one is interested in developing policy on diseases that are sexually transmitted – could not be more striking. In addition to an incomplete consideration of available scientific evidence, the process for naming political priorities in the Specific Populations Fund appeals to 'stakeholder consultation.' Yet as our experience in seeking funding from a community-based research fund illustrates, the invisible workings of HIV/AIDS institutions establish certain groups and constituencies as appropriate representatives of 'the community,' as stakeholders in the fight against AIDS. Populations such as bisexuals have not, historically, been well served (or even recognized) by existing actors within this field. Here again, we witness a certain tautology in thinking about, and responding to, HIV/AIDS: consultation with existing groups is done to determine priorities, and these groups then name the specific populations with whom they regularly work.

The Specific Populations Fund, then, provides a useful case study of the ways in which administrative procedures exclude certain groups and populations. The review of scientific evidence used to name priorities, as well as the consultation with relevant stakeholders, has made no sustained effort to consider the specific realities of bisexual men and women in Canada – despite the fact that bisexual men are figured to be vectors of infection among heterosexual women.

Conclusion

In this chapter, we have considered the invisible workings of institutions and how they frame the research that is done on HIV/AIDS – what is identified as a priority, what is funded, and why – as well as how research informs social policy and education. Referring back to our experiences in seeking funding for this research project, we teased out the manner in which misconceptions about bisexuality are pervasive and even inform the evaluative comments of scientific peer review committees. Furthermore, drawing on the framework known as institutional ethnography, we examined key documents in order to understand what kind of research is marshalled in social policies around HIV/AIDS in

Canada. Regulatory texts like *Leading Together* play an important role in determining future action in this domain: they coordinate the work of state institutions, services, and prevention. As we observed in our analysis of the Specific Populations Fund, the communities designated as priorities within regulatory texts are then renamed within subsidiary policy documents, such as funding application guidelines and orientations. Documents like *Leading Together* are more than mere reports. They organize the terrain in question, prescribing certain actions (i.e., prevention services for gay men) while foreclosing others (prevention services for bisexual men and women). In this regard, such documents coordinate ruling relations. We use this insight to expose how and why there is little or no mention of bisexuals within recent funding calls for national HIV prevention in Canada. Moreover, our work demonstrates how everyday people and communities are excluded from this research process, since it favours the voices of the existing HIV/AIDS agencies, which have done some excellent work but have also overlooked entire populations in responding to HIV. These elements – the ways in which misconceptions about bisexuality inform the grant evaluation process, the coordinating work done by a specific regulatory text, and the privileging of certain groups as 'community' – together provide an overview of how and why bisexuals have not even made it onto the map of HIV/AIDS research, policy, and education in Canada. This insight is as important as the results of our own empirical research, which we will present in subsequent chapters. Indeed, while initially we sought to obtain funding to conduct empirical research on bisexualities and HIV in Canada, our experiences in the granting application process helped us to think about the invisible, institutional ways in which research priorities are determined, as well as who gets left out of such an agenda. Moreover, these dynamics are complicated and need to be situated in much broader relations between community organizations and the state within a neoliberal context. Our discussion here explains the manner in which the grant evaluation of a community-based research committee is embedded within neoliberal social relations that position community organizations as service providers and that reduce political action to the lobbying of coalitions. Understanding how these dynamics function is crucial if we are to think critically about how to intervene in this situation.

This chapter has been concerned explicitly with questions of knowledge: what counts as knowledge, the research used to define priorities, the data that are disregarded, which actors are given a status of knowing, and the kinds of knowledge authorized within policy documents and regulatory texts in the field of HIV/AIDS in Canada. It is imperative to comprehend the complex dynamics at work in order to appreciate how much of our knowledge on HIV/AIDS is, in fact, circular. While such an insight is important, from the perspective of social action it remains insufficient. That is to say, it is not enough merely to understand how bisexuals have been excluded from HIV/AIDS research, policy, and education. One must also think about how to intervene in such a situation, and that is no small challenge!

If we have spent a great deal of time in this chapter outlining how and why bisexuals have been ignored, we now turn our attention to what can be done about it. How can we, in simple terms, put bisexuals on the map? What kind of knowledge is needed, and how do we go about gathering it? How do we imagine a research project that avoids so many of the pitfalls we have seen in thinking about, or eclipsing entirely, bisexual men and women? How can we move beyond mere critique (the exclusion of bisexuals from knowledge) to intervene concretely in the world, to create knowledge (finally) relevant to bisexual men and women? The following chapter answers these questions, through a detailed discussion of the methodology of our study.

3 Methods and Methodology: Designing an HIV Prevention Research Project Relevant to People Who Have Sexual Relations with Both Men and Women

The previous chapters examined questions of epistemology – how we know what we know, as well as the institutional relations between research, policy, and education. We demonstrated that there is a reciprocal relation between epistemology and methodology: the ideas and preconceptions we have about bisexuality inform, in turn, the questions researchers ask, how they code data, and the kind of evidence they then select for interpretation. With specific references to bisexuality, our discussion illustrated the limits and cultural bias of research in public health – studies that make 'ethnic culture' relevant in discussing the sexualities of non-white men but that ignore culture entirely when considering the sexualities of white men; investigations that underestimate the vulnerability of women to HIV and STDs – especially bisexual women – and exclude women from clinical trials and even the definition of disease itself; and projects that, in their coding of the data, quite literally make bisexuals disappear from view.

If our work has shown the weaknesses of public health research on bisexualities and HIV, what is the next logical step? How can one move beyond mere critique (important in itself) to generate knowledge that is grounded in people's everyday experience and is politically relevant? Given the lack of research and education adapted to the realities of bisexual men and women, how do we respond? What do we need to know? How do we go about getting that information? Why does it matter? Is there a way to link such research to action, and if so, how could that be done? In short, if the existing knowledge is biased and of limited use, how can we conceive and implement research otherwise?

It is, of course, in many ways easier to ask these questions than to answer them. Yet to not attempt an answer is a position that accepts the status quo – and that is an untenable position, in our view. For better or for worse, then, we set out to gather new kinds of information and to have such knowledge intimately connected to action. Our goal was to conduct research on bisexualities and HIV prevention that was specific and relevant, and that could in turn inform the development of appropriate educational materials. How we proceeded was, in many ways, in critical dialogue with what we considered to be the limits of the existing research and education. A more thorough consideration of how such limits helped frame our research is thus in order.

Our review of the scholarly literature and community education available on bisexuals and HIV demonstrated the ways in which social views shape the work of epidemiology. In this regard, our work is clearly informed by a sociological inquiry. Yet which kind of sociology ought to be privileged, since the field itself (like any discipline) is vast, with different currents, paradigm and internal dialogues? In broad terms, our theoretical and methodological reflections considered the ways in which bisexuals have been erased in public health research and education. Required, then, are research studies that give voice to such people. This reflects a commitment to a kind of social inquiry that is relevant to everyday people (Smith 1987; Smith 2005) – the men and women excluded from clinical definitions of disease, erased in the coding of data, underestimated in reviews of the scholarly literature, or just plain ignored. Since most studies make bisexuals disappear, there is an urgent need for critical research that includes them and ensures that their perspective is represented in the scholarly and public domains.

Interviews

We elected to gather information through interviews – a recognized method in qualitative research that is particularly useful in working with populations excluded from institutional life (Reinharz 1992). Interviews created an opportunity for men and women who had sexual relations with both men and women to talk about their specific needs. Given that we hoped this research could be used to develop educational materials, it was important to us from the beginning to ensure that we had captured the perspective and world view of these people. This focus on everyday people as a fundamental source of information is in line with the position articulated by Eric Mykalovskiy and Lorna Weir (2004), who argue that within the context of health research that relies on 'evidence-based medicine' (EBM), social scientists can make an important contribution to knowledge by considering the patient a site of EBM. To interview everyday men and women who have sexual relations with men and women about HIV prevention, then, positions their knowledge as relevant evidence in the formulation of health policy, services, and education.

But what should we ask people, assuming they will come and talk with us? It is all well and good to argue for the importance of asking everyday people about their needs, but at some level it also remains a bit vague. If the questions we pose are not especially relevant, we will have missed a unique opportunity to advance our knowledge in this domain. Here again, our reading of the limits of existing studies helped inform the content of our interviews. In our review of the literature, we noted that HIV research in the social sciences emphasizes behaviour with regards to sexual relations and drug use. Building on the knowledge generated with mainstream epidemiology, sociologists, sexologists, psychologists, and community health scholars inquire about the motivations and activities in which people engage. We examined an important limit of such an approach, however, in that it assumes people are comfortable speaking about their sexualities and drug use within a research-based context (even when confidentiality and/or anonymity is assured).

Furthermore, experts in the field now acknowledge that knowing about people's behaviour is not enough to understand how and why they decide to engage in high-risk activities. Data on behaviour in and of themselves do not inform the motivations that underlie decisions to adopt or avoid specific behaviour. In this regard, studies that focus on behaviour do not guarantee an immediate uptake of research findings: asking people about their sexual activities and risks cannot, at least in any straightforward way, tell you about the kinds of HIV education that should be developed.

Given these concerns, we decided to focus our interviews on HIV information. This is a frame that extends logically from our consideration of existing limits in the field: other researchers have not considered bisexual men and women in any meaningful manner and have assumed that most people will provide researchers with intimate details about their sexualities and drug use. Within the field, then, there is a dearth of information from people who have sexual relations with both men and women in general. Moreover – and this point is relevant to HIV research beyond the specific communities and realities of bisexual men and women – we have little knowledge about what people would like to see in HIV education. So asking everyday people not about their sex lives, but about the kinds of HIV education they need, shifts the focus radically. Such an approach puts the accent on their information needs – what kinds of prevention they need, how it should be presented, and where it should be available.

This focus on information, as opposed to behaviour, was fundamental to the results of our research as well as to the people who participated. Indeed, in our recruitment (more information on this subject below) and the actual conduct of the interviews, interviewers explained the terms and parameters of the study. When people called us to learn more about the project and possibly schedule an appointment for an interview, several expressed comfort and even relief that in the interviews they would not be asked to speak about their sexual lives in detail. This sentiment was well articulated by one participant, having spoken to a friend who had already participated in the study:

Parce que je trouve ça important aussi qu'on fasse ça, parce que je peux pas dire que moi ça me tentait, je l'ai vue ton annonce la semaine avant pis j'aurai pas appelé. Pis j'ai une amie qui est venue passer les tests de ça là, qu'est-ce qu'on fait, pis j'ai dit moi ça me tente pas. Pis là elle m'a dit mais c'est pas qu'est-ce que tu penses, elle dit c'est pas tes pratiques sexuelles en détail qu'ils veulent savoir.

(Because I find it important that we do that, like I can't say that I wanted to do it, I saw your ad last week and I would not have called. And I have a friend that came to do the interview and all that, and I said that I had no desire to do it. And she told me, 'Well it's not what you think.' She said, 'It's not detailed information about your sexual practices that they want to know.')

A certain discomfort with speaking about sexual behaviours was echoed by another interviewee:

It [the interview for this research] was pretty thorough without being too … you know, like details, details. You know what I mean? Like … 'cause I was kind of worried about that at first and I said that I don't want to get too, like, graphic about stuff. You know? 'Cause I'm just … that would make me uncomfortable.

These quotations underline an important methodological issue in public health research on HIV and STDs. Studies that emphasize sexual behaviour reflect a sample bias to the extent that they draw on a pool of participants who are comfortable providing information about their sex lives to a research team. By focusing on information, our study involved people who would not have participated in more traditional epidemiological, social scientific, and or sexological projects. Part of the reason the results of our study are new and innovative is, in our view, related causally to these methodological questions: our conceptual framework and orientation includes people who would choose not to participate in more traditional social science HIV research.

Interview Guide

The notion of information, as opposed to behaviour, was central to orienting our research, and specifically our interview questions. Indeed, we realized the difficulties in having people speak outside the standard 'tell us about your sexual behaviours in the past month' questionnaires. It took several drafts of our interview guide to ensure that we focused on information as opposed to behaviour – even though we remained critical of a behaviour-based approach, we found it more difficult in practice to formulate questions that moved beyond such a framework.

Our interviews were structured through an interview guide. This is a tool used in qualitative research that allows for overall coherence and structure for a series of interviews – each interviewee is asked the same questions in the same order. That said, an interview guide is just that – a guide to conducting the conversation (Reinharz 1992). It allows for some flexibility and openness, recognizing that research is, in its best possible sense, about discovery – and sometimes nuggets of information are buried within interviews that require further exploration and analysis. This approach to interviews is more flexible than a routinized, standardized questionnaire often used in social scientific research, which demands that each question be asked in the same way and the same order and allows no deviation from the protocol. Our approach was more organic: we ensured that the same general topics were covered during the interviews and generally were addressed in the same order. However, depending on the information provided by a participant at the beginning of a session, interviewers could move to a section further down the interview, or begin their analysis by asking someone to elaborate on something that stated early in the interview, or even in the moments immediately preceding the taped session.

We offer a summary of our interview guide here. We began with a collection of relevant demographic information – sex, age, income, education, ethnocultural background.[1] The interviews went on to inquire about how people access health information generally. Although the topic of our research was focused on HIV specifically, we elected to begin with a broader framework as a point of entry for gathering data. We felt that it would be useful to know, for instance, if most people first sought out health information via the Internet, hospital emergency rooms, or a health information line financed by the government (Info-santé). Having discussed access to health information and services generally, we moved on to inquire about people's knowledge and use of sexual health services. Importantly, here our questions remained in the third person – we asked, for example, what someone would do to get more information if friends thought they had an STD and needed information and possibly treatment. This framing in the third person represents one concrete instance where we tried to avoid a behaviour-based approach to research implicit in a question (for instance, 'Have you ever thought you had an STD? If yes, what did you do about it?'). By asking the question in the third person, individuals could respond in the hypothetical, without having to divulge information about their own sex life or sexual health history. Individuals reluctant to divulge their own sexual stories could easily remain in the hypothetical realm in their answer if they so chose – and many did just that. Moreover, such a framing centred the answer on health information and health services – which is precisely the research problematic we wished to understand more fully. We were (and are) interested in studying what kinds of HIV prevention people desire, and asking how they would access sexual health information and services is highly relevant therein. The answers tell us a great deal about the kinds of information people need, as well as where and how that information should be made available. The answers also inform us about gaps in the system. As we will see in the results and analysis section of this book, if people do not know where to find sexual health services, at some level their access to basic health services is compromised. Effective education needs to understand such problems in accessing services, and act accordingly (Namaste et al. 2007). We will develop this argument in greater depth later in this book.

We also asked people to tell us about their general impressions of the HIV education they had seen. What did they think about it? Did it appeal to them? Was it adapted to their needs? What were its strengths and weaknesses? Moreover, to try to get people to move beyond critique, we asked our participants to tell us what they thought was needed. What kind of information should be included for people that have sexual relations with both men and women? What format is the most appropriate?

We also gathered information about respondents' social networks. We certainly knew from our organizing work in bisexual and swinger communities that there is substantial diversity within such sites. We inquired about their friends and networks, social milieux, and the like. We also asked about their sexuality in very general terms (i.e., not an inventory of behaviours). We asked them to tell us about their sexualities in general – how they were organized, what they meant, if they would describe them with a particular word or name. Here, we wanted to ensure that we had a true diversity of respondents – if so, there would be great variation in how people located themselves in relation to sexuality (and indeed there was!). Importantly, this discussion focused on sexuality in general but avoided an identity-based frame of reference – that is, constant invocation of the term *bisexual*. We outline the importance of avoiding an exclusively identity-based approach to critical research on sexual health in more detail below.

Finally, we showed people two different HIV education advertisements that had been distributed in Québec within recent years (2000–4). Two posters were selected. The first was part of a national campaign directed to MSM, known as the Assumptions campaign. It reproduced an image of two men having anal sex, with the caption, 'Il me l'aurait dit s'il était séropositif. Il me l'aurait dit s'il était séronégatif. Comment fais-tu pour savoir?' (He would have told me if he was positive. He would have told me if he was negative. How do you know what you know?) The second example was a poster produced and distributed in Québec in bars, restaurants, and clubs. The poster contains images of headboards in a cemetery with the caption 'le sida tue toujours.' Our aim in showing these educational materials was not to conduct an official evaluation of these campaigns.[2] Rather, we sought to use these visual images and concrete examples as a way to stimulate reflection and discussion. This was often one of the most dynamic and animated aspects of the interviews. In some instances, people referred back to some of the points that they had made in a more general discussion of the limits of HIV education. In other instances, people who had little to say about HIV education when we raised the matter in the abstract actually had many things to say about these specific posters. We were interested in such information in order to consider the kinds of educational materials people do not like, as well as the kinds to which they would be more responsive.

The formal interviews we conducted were supplemented with observations from participation in relevant events (for example, a workshop organized by a local bisexual group, Bi Unité Montréal). We also made use of discussions and conversations with key people in the field – such as owners and managers of swinger establishments – to both gather and interpret data.

This interview guide, then, was designed to gather new and important information on the HIV prevention needs of people who have sexual relations with both men and women in Montréal. Moving beyond a behaviour-based inquiry, the research sought to garner new data useful to the development of educational materials. And importantly, this project was to consult everyday people themselves – giving them voice and ensuring that their world views and meanings are considered relevant evidence for health education and services.

Recruitment

Our review of the scholarly literature on bisexualities and HIV underlines the important distinction to be made between *behaviour* – the specific activities in which people engage – and *identity* – a particular name or category that one adopts. In the literature on MSM in particular, it is recognized that the importance of attending to behaviour cannot be underestimated. Yet our analysis of this scholarship, as well as the community education on which it is based, has contended that such an argument is more often rhetorical than not. HIV education and research is carried out under the banner MSM as a way to supposedly include all men who have sex with men, but in reality, this work speaks to gay men in particular. While we remain critical of such a rhetorical use of MSM as a category, we also recognize that the point being made is an important one: many individuals will engage in specific activities without attaching any label or identity to them. This insight is significant for the conceptualization of this project, with particular relation to questions of recruitment.

Within a public health context on HIV and bisexualities, questions of identity and behaviour are usually invoked to refer to men who have sexual relations with other men but who do not call themselves gay, or even bisexual. Careful attention needs to be paid, then, to strategies that do not privilege identity. While this frame of reference generally considers men only, it remains pertinent for the purposes of our study. Indeed, if we want to learn more about the needs of people who have sexual relations with both men and women in Montréal, to whom are we referring? Should we call these individuals 'bisexual,' even though many of them may not choose to name themselves as such? Should we focus on questions of behaviour? How can we ensure that a diversity of people who have sexual relations with both men and women would participate in our study? Where could we find them?

All of these questions – routine matters of ensuring the diversity of a sample population within research – helped us think about how to conceive this study in broad terms, and relatedly, how to recruit people. Yet we also confronted a lack of reflection on the concrete matter of recruitment in reaching individuals who refuse an identity (for example, non-gay MSM). Although public health research has a great deal to say about attending to behaviour rather than identity, it is relatively quiet on the specific modes in which one operationalizes it within research – MSM studies usually take place in sites associated with the gay male communities (bars, saunas), with little attention paid to the outreach and sampling strategies required to include non-gay MSM.[3] This absence merely reiterated the questions we had at the beginning: who do we mean when we say 'people who have sexual relations with men and women,' and how might we find them to inquire about their sexual health needs?

Our own knowledge and experience of organizing with bisexual communities was relevant here. In the late 1990s, three of the book authors (Tamara Vukov, Robin Williamson, and Viviane Namaste) had been involved in organizing a bisexual dance party in Montréal. At the time, there was no venue that was known specifically as an open dance establishment for meeting and/or cruising members of both sexes, and we organized to fill that gap. The parties, coincidentally named Soirée polyvalence, were held intermittently from 1999 to 2001. These events were successful on many levels: they drew upwards of two hundred people and garnered local and provincial media attention – articles appeared in *Voir* and *Montréal Mirror* (two free weekly newspapers), as well as *Clin d'Oeil*, a Québec women's magazine. These events were also unique, given the diversity of people present – attendees ranged in age from those in their twenties to others in their fifties, both men and women were present, some people were clearly politically involved bisexuals, people from many different ethnocultural communities came, and there were a significant number of swingers (couples who exchange sexual partners) present. The crowd was diverse, mixed, and fun! In our organizing efforts, we attributed this diversity to our specific outreach and promotion of the parties: our flyers advertised Soirée polyvalence as a night for 'bisexuals, the curious, and their friends.' Moreover, the media we received were in prominent, mainstream locations – getting the word out beyond a small population associated with a particular community (for instance, bisexuals who would align themselves with lesbian/gay communities).

This experience in community organizing for bisexuals in Montréal helped shape the terms of reference of this study. Having organized a party to which many different kinds of people came – under the banner 'bisexuals, the curious and their friends' – we wanted to interview people who were diverse in their age, gender, ethnocultural background, socio-economic status, and ways of living and articulating their bisexualities. Such an objective, of course, is easier said than done. But we had learned a few important lessons from organizing these events and were happy to implement them in the conception of this research.

We were interested in speaking with a variety of people, and so logically, we would need to have a variety of recruitment and outreach strategies. Securing the participation of a man who has sex with men, but who does not call himself gay, would likely require strategies and tactics different from those that recruited swinger couples. With this attention to diversity in mind, we thought about the research, and recruitment in particular, on three different 'networks' of people: bisexual women; swingers; and men and women who have sexual relations with both men and women, but without calling themselves bisexual. These 'networks' are not, of course, mutually exclusive: many women who identify as bisexual are also active in Montréal's swinger communities. Nor are such descriptions to be taken at face value: the point is not to offer an exhaustive description of different 'categories' of people with bisexual behaviour, as if that could even be possible (or desirable). Rather, we reasoned that if we recruited participants in three different ways (corresponding to the different 'networks' listed above), we would ensure participation from a diversity of people who live their sexualities in different ways. To speak, then, about such 'networks' of bisexuals is not to argue for the independent existence of such realities, but rather to be attentive to ways of gathering data that attempt to ensure a diverse sample population. In addition to this concern for diversity in our respondents, two additional criteria informed how we conceived of and recruited for the study: inclusion of women and acceptance of bisexuality in itself.

Our commitment to social inquiry on bisexualities and HIV that accounts for women's experiences emerges, in part, from our reading of the absences in this domain. Study after study on MSMs is published, but with virtually no reference to the female partners of such men. Moreover, our review of the epidemiological literature indicated the ways in which bisexual women are at greater risk for HIV than either lesbians or heterosexual women. Despite this empirical evidence, however, bisexual women have yet to be recognized as an at-risk population in discussions of women and HIV.

For all of these reasons, then, we were committed from the outset of this research to including women – and to ensuring that they were recruited in the first place. In a similar vein, our approach treats sexuality matter-of-factly. Since most other studies on bisexualities and HIV require people to 'prove' that they are 'really' bisexual, we decided not to proceed with a behaviour-based criterion for recruitment. Indeed, the last thing we wanted to do was ask people to justify or prove their sexualities. Rather, we would put the emphasis on their HIV information needs. Having considered these broader issues in how we conceptualize our work, we turn now to an overview of the recruitment strategies specific to each of the networks outlined above.

In our recruitment process overall, we made a deliberate decision to advertise for participants in mainstream venues and to avoid recruitment strategies that focused exclusively on social and/or community organizations. For example, although Montréal had a number of active community groups for bisexuals during the time we conducted this research, we concentrated our recruitment elsewhere. We were concerned about attracting potential respondents who identify clearly with the term *bisexual* if we recruited primarily through such groups – a strategy that would then underestimate or perhaps even ignore people who did not have an affiliation with that word. In this regard, we used small classified advertisements in a free weekly Montréal newspaper (*Voir*) as our primary means of recruitment. These advertisements were supplemented with outreach in certain public places and establishments.

Having conceived of different 'networks' of people with bisexual behaviour, we adapted our advertisements to specific realities. We began with outreach to bisexual women – our text sought out women who would respond to the term *bisexual women* and who were interested in speaking with us about their HIV prevention needs. This was the only recruitment advertisement we published that contained the term *bisexual*. Its use represents and reflects a certain reality – certainly, some men and women name themselves 'bisexual,' and the term has resonance with them. Yet our recruitment did not limit itself to such a name, in an effort to seek participation from a variety of individuals. In this regard, our classified advertisements for swingers asked respondents if they were swingers and if they had sexual relations with both men and women. Here, they did not need to name themselves 'bisexual' in order to participate in our inquiry. Our recruitment for swingers was supplemented by promotion in an electronic webzine for Québec swingers, as well as flyers distributed in some well-known swinger establishments, and a print advertisement published in an erotic magazine with significant swinger content and distributed free in Montréal-area sex shops. In the flyer and advertisement, two women and a man appear, alongside the caption, 'Are you interested in a threesome?' The accompanying text explains the purpose of the study and specifies that the research project is looking for individuals who have sexual relations with both men and women.

The final 'network' of people we set out to interview was those who had sexual relations with both men and women, without calling themselves bisexual. We did this section of the research last, in part because we anticipated some difficulties in finding such individuals. Yet since we had had enthusiastic response from the previous advertisements we had published in a free weekly newspaper, we decided to use this tactic again. We advertised, quite simply, for people who have sexual relations with both men and women to come and speak with us about their HIV prevention needs. The response to this particular advertisement was quite telling – and instructive. Respondents included both men and women (in roughly equal numbers), and significantly, many of them did not use the word *bisexual* to describe their sexuality and/or sexual orientation. For us, these data confirm the importance of careful attention to wording in study recruitment: we were able to gain participation from individuals who would not have granted an interview had we used the term *bisexual* exclusively. This sentiment was best captured by one of our interviewees, who made a point to tell us that he responded to our advertisement because of how it was worded:

> What I liked about the ad, it says, you know, 'people that have sex,' you know, 'with women and men.' They didn't say 'bisexual' or 'people, queer.'

This comment is revealing, because it reminds us of the doors that can be opened – or closed – depending on the words used in a recruitment advertisement. Not everyone we interviewed in the 'third network' of people refused to use the term *bisexual* categorically. Nevertheless, the information people shared with us suggests that our recruitment advertisement reached individuals who have sexual relations with both men and women, but who are not particularly invested in naming such an activity.

While the publishing of the recruitment advertisements was our primary means for getting people to participate, our attention to diversity in the sample population also meant we needed additional strategies. Once we had begun to schedule and conduct some interviews, then, we examined the demographic information in order to consider diversity. For example, if at one point we had interviewed only women under twenty, we would try to schedule additional interviews with women in an older age category, and any women under twenty who inquired about an interview were informed that at the current time, we were not accepting women of their age group. Or to take another example, we verified gender equity (more or less) among the swingers we interviewed, to ensure that we captured the perspective of both men and women. Our interviews were not, in this sense, 'first come, first served'; we struggled to ensure some amount of difference within our population. In certain cases, this required additional recruitment tactics: we sent out advertisements specific to lesbian/ gay/bisexual ethnocultural groups in our recruitment for bisexual women (one of the few instances in which we worked with organized groups), in an effort to ensure a good representation of people from ethnocultural communities in the sample. We also published recruitment advertisements in mainstream ethnocultural newspapers (hispanophone, anglophone black), and this tactic proved to be successful indeed – in fact, through an error in translation (the advertisement we had supplied in French was translated by one community newspaper into Spanish without our knowledge or request, and was published in Spanish only), a number of unilingual hispanophone respondents participated in our study. Since one of our team members was fluent in Spanish, this linguistic difference was easily accommodated. Sometimes, the 'mistakes' or errors that occur in research can be the best sources of data!

Overall, then, our strategies for recruitment reflected our commitment to ensure a diversity of respondents, as well as to avoid methodological and epistemological problems inherent in other public health research on HIV and bisexualities.

Statistical Overview of Study Respondents

For better or for worse, our recruitment was successful in soliciting the interest of potential participants. We had a constant and positive response to our advertisements and were rarely concerned about the possibility of no one coming forward to be interviewed! In the end, we interviewed a rather large group of people – eighty-seven in total. Analysis of the different components of the population reveals that it was relatively diverse:

- Sixty-six per cent of respondents were women, 34 per cent men. The over-representation of women in the total sample reflects the specific recruitment efforts, in that one 'network' of people identified was bisexual women.
- The age breakdown was relatively diverse: 5 per cent in the ten to nineteen age category; 39 per cent in the twenty to twenty-nine age group, and 26 per cent in the thirty to thirty-nine category. Polyvalence also succeeded in soliciting participation from older men and women: 21 per cent of respondents were aged forty to forty-nine, while 9 per cent of participants were between the ages of fifty and fifty-nine.
- Members of ethnocultural communities constituted 23 per cent of the sample population.
- French was the mother tongue for 74 per cent of respondents, English for 15 per cent, while 11 per cent of participants were allophone – having a mother tongue other than English or French.
- Fifty-eight per cent of interviewees declared an annual income of less than $20,000.

This statistical information provides some detail on the diversity and variation among the people who were interviewed in the *Polyvalence* study. In future chapters, we will examine what they identified as their needs in HIV prevention. For the moment, however, we need to underline two other important aspects embedded in the design and methodology of our project: community-based research and action research.

Community-Based Research and Action Research

This project is community-based, meaning that it emerged from the needs as articulated by a particular community and is conducted in collaboration with these people. A number of principles are especially relevant to the theory and practice of community-based research (CBR). We will focus on some of the most salient ideas here – relevance, ownership, and equity in partnership – and refer the reader to additional resources on CBR for further reading.[4] The idea of *relevance* is that the knowledge gathered is pertinent to the everyday lives and realities of the people concerned. It is a principle designed to ensure that research helps inform social change – that the questions asked are grounded in a firm understanding of people's needs (including the need for new knowledge), and that the answers to be put forward are connected to those same needs. An insistence on relevance within research rejects the generation of knowledge that responds to the institutional criteria of university-based scholars but does not help a community. Relevance means that the research question, process, and communication of results matter.

The concept of relevance in CBR is complemented by that of *ownership*: the knowledge generated within a research site belongs to its members. If a community organization helps a researcher gain access to the field in order to study young mothers and nutrition, the data and results are to be owned by both the researcher and community group. This principle avoids a hierarchy within the research process and underlines the fact that the contributions of community organizations are often central to effective research. This concept shifts a traditional relationship between scientists and community organizations, such as when community organizations provide access to the field, offer important contextual information required to make sense of data, and are given little or no credit as researchers in the final product.

The idea of ownership is closely linked to that of *equity in partnership*. According to this principle of CBR, all parties active in the research have equal weight, influence, and decision-making power, and this at all levels of the research – the initial question, recruitment, development of data collection tools, analysis, and sharing of research results. All members involved in research are equals in this regard, and all receive appropriate recognition – for example, their names on the final research reports, scientific articles and conference presentations.

These CBR principles informed this project from its initial stages: the research question itself emerged out of conversations among some of the authors of this book, in particular Viviane Namaste, Tamara Vukov, and Robin Williamson. How was it, we thought, that more than twenty-five years into an epidemic, there is no HIV information adapted to the lives of bisexual men and women? What explains the dearth of community education in this regard? (This book is, of course, a long answer to these questions!) We applied for funding to conduct research on this matter and were eventually successful. To ensure broader representation, we set up a community Advisory Committee, composed of ourselves as well as members of a local bisexual association (Bi Unité Montréal) and a local HIV/AIDS group (GAP-Vies). Advisory Committee members were active in the research process – they reviewed drafts of the interview guide, for example, and made suggestions for improvements. One such suggestion was to include a section where we showed participants previous HIV posters, as a way to get them talking about what they did and did not like. We incorporated this feedback, and indeed it turned out to be one of the most important elements of the interviews, providing us with a wealth of data. This example provides a useful illustration of how beneficial CBR can be – members can identify needs that might be overlooked by a researcher working in isolation. Advisory Committee members were also involved in recruitment, suggesting places to locate potential interview subjects and discussing the advantages and disadvantages of conceptualizing the project in relation to three 'networks' of people. Furthermore, Advisory Committee members were involved in the data analysis. For reasons of time and efficiency, the initial summary of the data analysis was done by the principal investigator and the paid research team – we had the time to read through eighty-seven interviews and look for common themes. Once we prepared a summary document, it was presented to other Advisory Committee members – who offered critical feedback and asked questions as to how we could use this information in a positive way. Finally, all members of the project have their names on all documents such as publications and scientific conference presentations. This practice recognizes the involvement of all members.

If the above description illustrates how this project adheres to the principles of CBR, it is also necessary to outline the practice of action research and discuss how this paradigm informs this particular project. Action research is a specific tradition of gathering knowledge that is designed to yoke knowledge and action (Stringer 1999). Sometimes referred to as participatory action research (PAR), this approach is especially popular in certain academic disciplines – education, communication studies, international development, sociology, and women's studies. (This list is, of course, not exhaustive.) PAR shares with CBR a commitment to recognizing and valuing the involvement of everyday people in knowledge production: the meaningful participation of individuals and communities outside the university is central to this practice. Yet PAR also advocates a specific approach to knowledge that may or may not be shared by CBR, and that is an insistence on action.

Various traditions and streams within PAR offer different ways to conceive of this relation between knowledge and action. In projects undertaken in a school, for example, the research may be designed to improve curriculum development. Such a model does not advocate for action directly in the research – the point is not to offer a new curriculum, but first to study what does and does not work (and why), in order to then use this information in the development of new pedagogical materials. Other models in PAR advance a position in which action holds a more central role and in which action is itself incorporated into a research project. Regardless of the particular tradition or stream within PAR, all PAR projects share a commitment to thinking through how knowledge and action connect. PAR is a framework in which knowledge and action inform each other (Herr and Anderson 2005; Stringer 1999).

Our research project draws inspiration from PAR in that we were committed to action on bisexualities and HIV. In setting out to do this work, we were not interested in only identifying the need for HIV education that was adapted to individuals who have sexual relations with both men and women. We could have, for instance, quite easily designed a research study in which we considered the absence of HIV material in this domain. Yet such an approach was unsatisfactory for us – we were already well aware of such a gap in resources. We needed to understand how and why such an absence has persisted for so long. And perhaps more importantly, we needed to think very concretely about what could be done. Was there a way in which our research could assist in getting relevant educational materials out into the public domain? Here, the tradition of action research gave us inspiration and direction. This project was conceptualized in dialogue with the idea that the generation of knowledge should be linked to action. More specifically, the project was designed so that the research process itself would include action. We were not interested in offering a merely descriptive analysis of the situation, to spend tens of thousands of dollars in order to reach what was to us a rather banal conclusion: 'There is a need for HIV education that is adapted to the sexual lives of people who have sex with both men and women.' Rather, we wanted our project to *do something*, to actually intervene in the current situation. In this regard, we designed a project whose goal was to create appropriate HIV educational materials for men and women with bisexual behaviour in Montréal. This focus on action oriented our work – the data gathered, the analysis of results, and how such findings could be used. In very simple terms, the idea behind this project was to ask everyday people who have sex with both men and women what they would like to see in HIV education, and then to go about creating some of those resources.

The process of developing these educational materials occurred at the Advisory Committee level. Once we had considered the data from the interviews, we sat down to consider how one could translate the findings into concrete educational materials. At times this process was straight-forward – people suggested, for instance, that posters include both a website and a phone number, and so it was relatively easy to ensure this was accomplished. In other instances, however, it was more challenging to translate the findings. In our interviews with women in particular, we found that most women did not have access to good information about the risks of HIV and STD transmission between women. Indeed, many of our participants had more questions than answers in this regard! Such a finding poses a challenge for the development of a poster, given that HIV education usually tells people what specific behaviours to avoid and/or how to minimize their risk. What could we say about woman-to-woman transmission? Use a dental dam or latex barrier every time you have oral sex with a woman? If this was necessary, why are there no HIV mate-rials directed to heterosexual men that outline the importance of this practice (Gorna 1996)? In the case of women-to-women transmission, we found that we had many more questions than answers. Ultimately, it was in fact these questions that informed the development of our posters. Since everyone we talked to had poor information on this sub-ject, we began by asking this precise question, asking readers/viewers if they know the risks of HIV and STD transmission between women, and providing two different means for them to get more information in this regard. The details we present here underline our commitment to an action-oriented process: to take the results of our interviews and cre-ate meaningful education materials. In this manner, our research project sought to connect knowledge and action.

Conclusion

This chapter has provided an overview of the decisions we made about how to conceive and orient our project, how to gather data and analyse them, and how to connect this knowledge to action. These specific choices in method – the concrete techniques of gathering information – are in turn linked to the broader epistemological questions we considered previously in our review of the limits of public health research on bisexualities and HIV, as well as our examination of the institutional workings of HIV/AIDS research and policy. In that review, we demonstrated the ways in which bisexual men and women are written out of public health research and education. Given such an omission, this project has made careful and considered choices about how to go about acquiring and making use of new information. We propose a framework that breaks ground with many of the traditional ways of thinking about bisexualities and HIV: focusing on information rather than behaviour, ensuring that women are (finally) included, accepting people's bisexuality when they state it and refusing to make them justify or prove its validity, using varied recruitment strategies to ensure a diverse sample population, avoiding an identity-based logic in inquiry, gaining information through interviews, incorporating community members through all aspects of the research process, and building an action component into the research design itself. In all of these ways, this research seeks to gain new insight into the current gaps in HIV education for men and women with bisexual behaviour, as well as to intervene in the situation.

Having outlined our specific methodological choices, as well as their connection to matters of epistemology, we are ready to present the results of our study – to consider the kinds of HIV education materials desired by our participants, and to discuss how we used these results in the development of prevention posters. Finally, we can allow bisexual men and women to speak for themselves.

4 'The Message Is Ugly, You Know?' Limits of HIV Education in Québec

In the previous chapters, we examined some of the main problems with knowing bisexualities, and with doing empirical research on them. This chapter shifts the focus somewhat, insofar as we consider the experiences and opinions of men and women who have sexual relations with both sexes with respect to HIV education and services. Whereas previous chapters outlined the epistemological and methodological issues at stake, this chapter brings forth the voices of the participants in our study.

Some of the results presented here are specific to this population – for example, interviewees explain the ways in which current campaigns do not give adequate attention to bisexual realities. Yet in other instances, the results are relevant for developing effective HIV/AIDS education more generally, such as when interviewees remind academic researchers to avoid a technical vocabulary that is quite specific to public health (e.g., the term *seropositive*). In these different ways, then, the research to be presented in this chapter offers insightful and compelling ways to reconsider how we go about doing HIV prevention more broadly. Given the dearth of empirical studies that begin their inquiry by asking people about the kind of HIV education they would like to see, we feel that the findings of this study are important. They offer a useful point of departure to develop campaigns specific to bisexual men and women, but also to rethink more generally the way we go about doing HIV prevention work.

The data that follow are taken from the empirical interviews conducted, as well as from observations in bisexual and swinger milieux. The networks of people outlined in chapter 3 are represented here (bisexual women, swingers, and people who have sexual relations with both men and women, but without calling themselves bisexual), with an analysis of a context specific to a certain milieu when relevant. Thus, some of the results here are common across the networks studied – for instance, the ways in which HIV education is not adapted to the realities of people who have sexual relations with both men and women, since it often ignores partners of both sexes. In other instances, however, the findings are specific to a certain milieu. This is the case, for example, in our research with swingers, in which they talk about the way that HIV education does not address the specific need to use a new condom with each new act of penetration, and each sexual partner, within group sexual relations. In all instances, the results presented here provide fresh insight into what everyday people think about the kind of HIV education available in Québec, as well as what could be done to improve the situation. One final note concerning the data presented: the quotations are from both men and women. However, our findings indicate that women in particular experience tremendous difficulties in accessing relevant information and services in the field of HIV. Given the severity of the difficulties presented, as well as the frequency with which such problems were cited in our interviews, we have elected to devote the next chapter specifically to women's experiences in HIV education and services. While this chapter does not expand in detail on women's lives and perceptions, it offers an overview of the difficulties in accessing information and services more generally. This background will facilitate comprehension of the manner in which such problems are further gendered – a topic to be addressed in greater depth in chapter 5.

The present chapter has two broad objectives: to identify the limits of existing HIV education and services, as expressed by participants in our study, and to offer concrete solutions to improve the kind of prevention information to be offered. These two objectives are, of course, complementary. An identification of the problems is central, because as we have seen in previous chapters, there remains an urgent need for systematic documentation of the problems bisexuals face in accessing HIV education and services.[1] This research represents the first large-scale study of this problematic in Canada.[2] Yet documentation of problems is insufficient in itself, at least if we are interested in connecting knowledge to action in a dynamic way. In this regard, we ask people what should be done about the problems they face, and present their suggestions. In chapter 7, we discuss how our research project incorporated these suggestions within the action components of this initiative.

The quotations and experiences cited below offer an overview of the ways in which HIV education is not adapted to the needs of men and women who have sexual relations with both sexes. Yet these data also tell us how and why certain people are excluded from institutions. This focus on institutions, then, remains a common thread with the previous chapters. Whereas our work up until this point has examined the specific theoretical, research, policy, and administrative ways that exclusion is structured in institutions, this chapter outlines what the consequences of such exclusion can be: lack of knowledge, total absence of information, outright refusal of services, and violation of human rights. Having outlined such difficulties, we then draw on the voices of our participants to suggest ways in which the current situation can be improved. In so doing, we hope that this research offers more than a critical regard of how exclusion is organized in and through institutions, as well as how it is experienced. We hope that this research can provide new ways of thinking about doing the mundane work of HIV prevention.

One final issue needs to be addressed before we present the results. The participants cited here identify specific information needs that they have in HIV prevention and services. In this instance, information refers to the specific data and concrete details about how to protect oneself and one's partner, and or how to find a local service for an HIV test. The particular and technical aspect of *information*, however, is intimately related to broader questions of *knowledge*. When the men and women interviewed state the need for educational materials that are relevant to them and their sexual partners, they cite a gap in information available. Yet at the same time, they raise an important critique of how information is made available in the first place – the decisions made behind the scenes about what the specific content of HIV prevention will be, the people to be targeted, and/or where information will be distributed. In this regard, the particular matter of information is connected to knowledge – which is to say, what counts as relevant data to be known and distributed, what kinds of details are considered essential to our understanding, and which ones are absent. As a concept, knowledge involves a certain level of abstraction and in addition is situated within certain social relations (Mort and Smith 2009). Our discussion of the knowledge of mainstream epidemiology presented in chapter 2 illustrates how the normative social relations of sexuality influence how researchers code and organize categories of sexuality within public health research. (Institutional ethnography, of course, is part of a broader project of the sociology of knowledge: see Smith [1987; 2006].) Yet information, despite having less abstraction and a more direct, referential relation to the social world, is also situated within specific social relations. Indeed, the specific content of information that circulates within the world, as well as the kinds of information unavailable, needs to be understood as located within specific knowledge frameworks themselves determined by larger social relations. Thus, the challenge is not simply to take the content of information at face value, but rather to understand the ways in which such content is imbricated in social relations, which are pervasive and often invisible. To extend this argument further, to inquire about information needs (such as those of bisexuals vis-à-vis HIV prevention) opens the possibility of a critique of existing knowledge frameworks and the institutional relations that support them. The information gaps identified by participants should thus be examined as created by organizing our HIV/ AIDS knowledge in a particular way. Throughout the presentation of research results (chapters 4, 5, and 6), we will underline the ways in which the voices of participants speak to more than the need for specific content with regards to HIV prevention. They offer a compelling analysis of the social organization of knowledge itself.

Information

Our study began with a basic premise: to ask people who have sexual relations with both men and women to tell us about their needs in HIV education. This necessarily requires having them speak about the information available to them and their reflections on its strengths and weaknesses. The participants in this research identified a number of difficulties with accessing information about HIV and sexually transmitted diseases. For some people, there was an utter absence of information:

> Il y a pas, il y a pas, il y a pas de publicité, il y a pas de, de, d'informations … Comment gérer des comportements dans ces moments de, MTS, j'ai un ami voilà deux semaines qui a été pris avec des morpions. Ça été la panique totale … La panique totale, c'est ça. Une chance que, il y avait des amis qu'on connaissait un peu ça pis qu'on a dit, ben oui, mais, cette personne-là aurait pu se suicider ce soir-là … Parce que, elle est pas au courant. Tsé, les gens, tsé je veux dire, je veux dire, des morpions ça existe. Jamais on n'a vu d'annonce publicitaire. Jamais on a vu de flyers de passés sur ça.

(There is no publicity, there is no information. How to behave in these times, STDs, I have a friend who, just two weeks ago, had crabs. It was absolute panic. Absolute panic, that's it. Good thing that there were some friends who knew a little bit about that, because, well yes, that person could have committed suicide that night. Because she was not aware. You know, people, I mean, crabs, they exist. We have never seen an ad about that. We've never seen pamphlets passed around about that.)

While this interviewee cites a complete lack of information, others offer a somewhat more nuanced approach. They note that information on HIV and STDs is available in a broad sense, but it remains quite general.

Euh, je suis certaine que je vais mettre cinq, six, huit personnes devant moi puis je vais leur demander de m'expliquer c'est quoi la syphilis … la plupart savent pas. Le monde, tout le monde a entendu ce mot-là, tout le monde en a parlé, a entendu parler des morpions, tout le monde a entendu parler de l'herpès. mais c'est quoi? Ça s'attrape comment? C'est quoi incubation? C'est quoi la … Personne sait ça.

(Well, I'm sure that if I put five, six, eight people in front of me and I ask them what syphilis is, most of them don't know. People, people have heard of that word, everybody's talked about it, has heard about crabs, everyone has heard about herpes. But what is it? How can one catch it? What's the incubation period? Nobody knows that.)

Il y a un énorme travail à faire puisque les gens restent quand même un petit peu ignorants de tous les … tous les envers de la médaille, ou même les symptômes qu'ils peuvent dire à quelqu'un écoute il faudrait peut-être que t'ailles consulter. Il y a des gars, comme un médecin m'expliquait, qui peuvent traîner ça pendant un an de temps sans savoir qu'ils ont une MTS, ils vont le donner à quelqu'un d'autre sans savoir … Donc c'est toutes des choses qu'on est peut-être pas assez sensibilisé à ce niveau-là, aux symptômes réels de ces maladies-là.

(There is a very big job to be done, because people remain nonetheless a bit ignorant of all the … all the other sides of the coin, or even the symptoms, so that they can say to someone, 'Listen, you had better get checked out.' There are guys, like a doctor explained to me, that can carry that for a year without realizing they have an STD. They are going to give it to others without knowing. So it's all these things about which there isn't enough education, real symptoms of these diseases.)

These quotations underline the fact that, while there may be some general discussion of sexual health in Québec society, specific information about the symptoms and treatment of STDs is generally less well known.

Incomplete understandings of disease symptoms and treatments reflect not a complete absence of information, but the fact that much of the information that is available is contradictory. The participants we interviewed contended that one of the biggest challenges in access to sexual health information is being able to evaluate such information properly:

> Parce que je veux dire souvent, le, l'information est contradictoire … Il y a énormément d'informations aujourd'hui. C'est très facile d'en trouver de l'information. Mais laquelle est bonne? … C'est ce qui est le plus difficile. Je veux dire, sur Internet, tu tapes n'importe quel mot, ça te sort trois millions cinq cents milles quelque chose fichiers. Il y en a de l'information. Mais souvent il faut lire plusieurs aspects pour se faire une bonne idée c'est quoi du problème.

> (Because I mean, often, the information is contradictory. There is so much information today. It's really easy to find information. But which one is the right one? That's more difficult. I mean, on the Internet, you type in any word, you get three million five hundred thousand dossiers. Information is there., but often you have to read many aspects to get a good idea of what the problem is.)

Difficulties in evaluating sexual health information are exacerbated in the era of the Internet. Participants noted that the problem is not always finding information, but finding information that is relevant, accessible, and comprehensive.

> Mais c'est ça, si la personne ne sait pas où aller chercher de l'information pis euh elle tape le mot *Sida* euh sur le, l'internet, la personne elle va revirer folle.

> (But that's it, the person doesn't know where to get information, and she types in the word *AIDS* on the Internet, the person is going to go crazy.)

One interviewee recounts her experience in trying to locate information about chlamydia on the Internet:

> Ben, ok, je vais t'expliquer de quoi de réel qui est arrivé hier. Je cherchais euh ... parce qu'il y a quelqu'un que je connais qui a la chlamydia. Fait que elle là, elle a pas Internet. Donc, je suis allée sur le site, j'ai fait Chlamydia. Euh, j'ai trouvé des choses qui m'ont amenée à d'autres choses. En tous cas j'avais comme dix fenêtres ouvertes, pis il y avait rien qui répondait à ma question ... Internet, j'ai fait chlamydia, je suis allée sur Toile du Québec, je suis allée sur euh, euh ... MSN, je suis allée sur Canoë ... Tsé, il y avait pas chlamydia: définition, symptômes ... Tsé, c'est ça je voulais moi.

> (OK, I'll explain to you what actually happened to me yesterday. I was looking, because I know someone who has chlamydia. So she ... she doesn't have Internet. So I went onto the site, I put in 'chlamydia.' I found things that led me to other things. In any case I had like ten windows open, but nothing that answered my question. Internet, I put in 'chlamydia,' I went on the Toile du Québec, I went on MSN, I went on Canoë. You know, there wasn't chlamydia: definition, symptoms. That's what I wanted.)

This quotation reveals one of the main difficulties people have in locating information about HIV and STDs. The issue is not finding information per se – that is easily done when one has access to a computer and the Internet. But such an operation does not guarantee that one can locate information that is pertinent and easily comprehensible. These difficulties, then, suggest that to think critically about providing people with HIV and or STD information is a matter more complex than simply ensuring that the information is publicly available. To be sure, there is a need to ensure that such information is out there and is presented in an accessible format. Yet the participants in our study also contend that they need a way to evaluate the information with which they are presented.

These difficulties in evaluating and accessing information were one of the most important recurrent themes within this research project and one evidenced in each of the three different networks under consideration. Indeed, whether the person interviewed was a suburban swinger, a political bisexual, or just an everyday person who likes to have orgasms with both men and women, interviewees consistently remarked on their difficulties in obtaining adequate sexual health information. These reflections raise important questions not only of the content of sexual health information, but also of its distribution and organization. For many people interviewed, the challenge is not so much finding information, but rather being able to locate accurate information that one can evaluate critically. As such, participants raise questions about how information is organized, about the specific frameworks of knowledge that underline HIV prevention. In particular, they question the assumption that the challenge of HIV prevention is simply to provide information, and they suggest that successful education must also facilitate a context for people to make sense of such information. Their experiences underline the knowledge components of HIV prevention, offering a critique of the ways in which current paradigms are inadequate to the complexity of the social world.

In the section that follows, we focus our attention more closely on the specific content of HIV education. We consider both the problems identified by our participants within the campaigns (specifically a lack of information adapted to their sexual lives), as well as the concrete suggestions that they put forward in order to provide more meaningful and comprehensive HIV and STD prevention information.

Current HIV Campaigns: Shooting Ourselves in the Foot?

In our interviews, we asked people what they thought about existing HIV educational campaigns. As outlined in chapter 3, we showed them examples of some specific campaigns that had been conducted in Québec as one way to generate feedback and to have their comments grounded in the concrete and everyday. We also asked people about the kinds of information they need and how it should be delivered. The results of this research are important – in terms of documenting the ways that education has excluded the realities of people who have sexual relations with both men and women, and in making some critical suggestions for how to conceive and implement HIV education (regardless of a specific community targeted).

'The Message Is Ugly, You Know?': Beyond Fear-Based HIV Campaigns

One of the most salient findings of our research was the tone of HIV education. There was no unanimity on how to frame advertisements.

Some participants recognized the importance of getting people's attention. Thus dramatic advertisements were applauded:

C'était une bonne publicité. Très bonne euh … accrocheur comme j'ai dit tantôt, mais euh … moi je pense c'est la meilleure publicité qui a été fait à date pour montrer dans un cercueil, oui ça mène jusque là.

(It's a good ad. Very good, it really grabs you, like I said earlier, but … me, I think that it's the best ad to date to show that a coffin, yes, it leads there.)

R: Yes. Excellent! This, I would put up everywhere. This, I like. Yes. It's still there. Excellent. This is the best thing I've seen so far.
Q: Yeah?
R: Oh yeah. This is heavy.
Q: What do you like?
R: The graves. That if you don't take care, that's where you'll end up. This is very serious. This is very, very special. Yeah. Yeah, excellent.

While certain people interviewed appreciated education that underlined the seriousness of HIV, many more we interviewed objected to campaigns organized around the notion of fear, and particularly the fear of death.

Q : Pis est qu'il y a des approches que t'as vues que t'aimes moins ou tu penses marchent moins bien comme stratégies de parler aux gens.
R : Dans, ben dans la peur, c'est sûr, la peur là … il faut que ça t'atteint euh … mais il faut pas que ça te fasse peur. Parce que souvent ça va avoir faire peut-être même le contraire ou euh … tu vas changer, c'est pas intéressant, tu vas changer de poste. Si tu te sens agressé là, tu sais, tu te sens inquiet, tout ça la, tu sais c'est … Non, c'est pas une bonne approche ça.

(Q: And are there approaches that you have seen that you like less, or that are less effective as strategies to reach people?
R: Well, in fear, for sure, fear, it can get your attention. But it shouldn't make you afraid. Because often it is going to possibly have the opposite effect. You're going to change, it's not interesting, you're going to change the channel. If you feel attacked, you know, you're worried, all of that, you know. No, that's not a good approach.)

Q : Et quelles sont tes impressions de l'info sur la prévention de VIH qui est disponible?

R : Ben moi je trouve que c'est trop agressif … Tu sais, au lieu de dire, comment je pourrais dire ça? Tu sais. Au lieu de dire que tu peux mourir à long terme, eux-autres ils disent euh … « tu vas mourir euh [*rires*] finalement là » tu sais.

(Q: And what are your impressions of the HIV prevention information that is available?
R: Well, I find it too aggressive. You know, instead of, how can I say that? You know, instead of, you can die in the long term, they say, 'You're going to die.' You know.)

C'est trop laid [annonce « le sida tue encore »]. Pis je parle pas juste laid de l'image … le message est laid, tsé.

(It's too ugly [the ad, 'AIDS still kills']. And I'm not just talking about an ugly image. The message is ugly, you know.)

R : Mais je suis, je trouve que c'est pas tellement de l'information, c'est plus une euh … une campagne de propagande.
Q : Oui. Ok. Oui. Pourquoi vous, vous … vous dites que c'est une campagne de propagande, pourquoi?
R : Ben je dis que c'est un peu plus, ben de, de jouer sur la, sur la peur des gens … Que de jouer sur l'information.

(R: But I, … I find it's not really information, it's more of a propaganda campaign.
Q: Yes. OK. Yes. Why, you say that it's a propaganda campaign. Why?
R: Well it's a little more, well, to play on the fears of people, as opposed to giving information.)

For many participants, fear-based campaigns actually backfire, to the extent that the reader/viewer rejects entirely the message advanced:

Mais pas nécessairement que ce soit euh … tsé comme euh … percutant mais que ça te donne mal au c'ur de regarder l'annonce là. Tsé comme euh … tsé le sida c'est un borderline là, tsé. Le truc euh des cercueils là … Tsé pas des, des trucs euh … ça là j'haïs ça là. Tsé des … que tu vois quelqu'un qui a le cancer qui est tout … euh le sida qui est tout euh … tsé pas, pas des choses euh vulgaires pis qui, qui rabaissant euh l'homme euh avec un grand 'H' là. Il faudrait que ce soit plus de la sensibula … sensibilisation pis des, des bonnes photos là. Pas d'affaires de … « On veut vous, vous écoeurer pis faites attention, pis on veut vous faire peur parce que attention, il y a la maladie », parce que moi je pense pas que ça marche ça.

(Well, not that it necessarily be, you know, like shocking but it makes you sick to look at the ad. You know, like AIDS it's borderline. This thing with the coffins, you know, things like that, I hate that. You know, you see someone who has cancer, AIDS, who is all … You know, not vulgar things, or things that denigrate someone. There has to be more education, and nice photos. Not these, 'We want to piss you off, and pay attention, and we're going to bother you because, careful, there's this disease,' because me, I don't think that that works.)

R: 'Cause I also don't think the fear of death campaigns … are any good either.
Q: What don't you like about them? Or what do you think is ineffective?
R: Well they take you to the point where you never want to have sex again … and then … in order to have sex again … you completely ignore everything you've heard.

Such a critical perspective on HIV education, in which a message motivated by fear is set aside or outright rejected by everyday people, is in fact supported by scientific evidence. Studies in health promotion indicate that fear-based attempts to induce behaviour modification are unsuccessful (Gagnon, Jacob, and Holmes 2010; Tripp 1988).

Several interviewees in our study offered a nuanced reading of HIV campaigns that actually create confusion about how HIV is transmitted. By relying on a fear of sex and death, according to these participants, fear-based campaigns equated sexual relations per se, rather than *unprotected sexual relations*, with risk:

This to me, is the kind of ad that would instil panic. Not so much the desire to look out and find. I mean, it's great for shock value. If it gets people talking and gets journalists writing about the new campaign and therefore leads to putting out information … super cool … You know? But I mean, equating going to bed with death sounds like a pretty judgmental kind of message … You don't die because you have sex.

Ça fait peur pour la sexualité des gens. Ça leur fait plus peur d'avoir des relations sexuelles que d'avoir … des relations protégées puis … c'est ça.

(It creates fear about people's sexuality. It makes them more afraid to have sexual relations than to have protected relations … that's it.)

C'est vraiment clair. Le message est là. Sauf qu'encore, ils disent que ... ils disent pas tout qu'est-ce qu'il y a avant [*ricane*]. C'est tout de suite, euh le sida ça tue. Tu fais l'amour, tu meurs. C'est comme ça un peu, tu sais, pis c'est pas ça exactement ça ... C'est le sida qui tue ok, mais c'est les relations non-protégées, ça devrait être plus dans ce sens-là.

(It's really clear. The message is there. Except that, they say that, they don't talk about everything before [*laughs*]. It's right away, 'AIDS kills.' You make love, you die. It's a little bit like that, you know, and it's not exactly like that. OK, it's AIDS that kills, but it's unprotected sexual relations, it should be more in that sense.)

When asked about what they thought of the HIV campaigns they had seen recently, and when presented with some sample advertisements, the majority of participants in our study offered a negative evaluation of a fear-based approach to education. In addition to such general comments, our respondents provided a detailed and compelling analysis of the ways in which the content of existing HIV education did not address the complexities of their lives as people who have sexual relations with both men and women.

Lack of Information concerning Both Male and Female Partners in Existing Campaigns

Most HIV campaigns our respondents had seen were directed to either gay men or to heterosexuals. They had not come across education that integrated sexual relations with both men and women within the message and framework.

Encore là on montre l'homosexualité, ça fait que j'aurais peut-être changé le phénomène, j'en aurais mis trois, deux gars avec une fille en avant ou au milieu d'eux autres comme juste pour le fait ... parce que encore là on est pas rejoint, on est pas ciblé là-dedans dans cette pub-là, c'est sûr et certain que oui quand on se sent concerné, mais sinon, si je regarde ça, je me sens pas concernée, c'est deux gars. Ça fait que je pense que ... c'est ça que j'expliquais tantôt, de rajouter des fois une troisième personne ou des choses comme ça va faire comme okay, oui, je suis pas homosexuelle mais j'ai quand même des relations comme ça, donc je suis à risque moi aussi.

(Once again it's homosexuality that is represented. Me I would shake it up, I would put two, three guys with a woman in front or among them, just to … because once again we don't reach the target in this ad, for sure the target it reached if one feels concerned, but otherwise, I look at that, I'm not concerned, it's two men. So I think that, it's what I was saying before, to add a third person or things like that that will make it like, OK, I'm not homosexual but I have relations like that, so I'm at risk too.)

Ben si je vois une annonce sur les homosexuels, je me sens pas … C'est comme si je me sens pas visé là, tu sais.

(Well, if I see an ad for homosexuals, I don't feel … It's like I'm not concerned, you know.)

But I guess stuff is still talked about in terms of gay and straight. I'll constantly hear about how straight women … contracting HIV or whatever. And so I'm just, like, well, I'm sort of half a straight woman, but I don't know if I really see myself as a straight woman, or like, my friends who have sex with guys and who are women would never see themselves as straight. I don't know.

The absence of women in most campaigns was cited as a severe limitation, and this subject will be addressed in greater depth in the next chapter. The above quotations are relevant to these matters of gender. When an advertisement contains only images of men, the men and women we interviewed did not see it as one that was targeted to bisexuals. This insight suggests that, notwithstanding a discourse and public health funding of MSM initiatives, HIV education that includes only men's bodies does not reach non-gay-identified men who have sexual relations with men. Such a limitation is further evidenced by the following quotations from men who were reacting to a specific advertisement showing a visual representation of anal sex (the Assumptions campaign).

Je va plus m'en, je va plus te, te … te dire euh qu'est-ce que j'aime pas. C'est, c'est les photos ici. Il y a … parce que moi je vois euh comme, comme si on est … on, on, on utilise … quand on met du sexe là, on utilisait la'tout le temps l'encu …, l'enculage là … Je veux dire euh … il y a d'autres positions que ça là … Pas à cause qu'on est deux hommes qu'il y a pas rien d'autre que.

(I'm going to tell you what I don't like. It's these photos here. Because me, it's like when we use … when sex is put there, it's always anal sex that is used. And I mean, there are other positions than that! It's not because we're two men that there isn't something else.)

R : Ça j'aime pas beaucoup ça.
Q : Mm-hm. Pourquoi?
R : Parce que moi première des choses, quand j'ai une relation homosexuelle, euh j'ai … jamais de relation comme ça … Ça, ça a de l'air d'un homme qui est en train d'enculer un autre homme. Ben [*ricane*] j'aime pas ça … J'aime pas ça.

(R: I don't like that very much.
Q: Mm-hm. Why?
R: Well, first of all, when I have a homosexual relation, I don't ever have a relation like that. It looks like a man who is fucking another man. Well [*laughs*], I don't like that, I don't like that.)

Both of these men offer important insight into the ways in which HIV education can implicitly exclude certain viewers or targeted people, depending on its content. Visual iconography that represents only anal sex, according to our respondents, sends a clear message that the education is directed to gay men in particular. Effective strategies to reach non-gay men, then, need to consider representing a diversity of bodies – including women's bodies – and sexual practices.

Our respondents signalled that current education does not consider their sexual lives in a number of ways. We have considered two major limitations in this regard: providing visual representation and practical information about both male and female partners, and offering images that appeal to the diversity of sexual practices for bisexual men and women (not limiting themselves, for example, to anal sex). An additional weakness in the content of HIV and STD education as identified by our participants concerns multiple partners. This issue was identified in particular by the swingers we interviewed but was also raised throughout our different interviews. The people we spoke with offer compelling critiques of current HIV education, which generally speaks of sexual relations between two people. Yet there are specific concerns raised when one considers having multiple partners, perhaps especially multiple partners at the same time – as in the context of swinging and / or group sex. The following quotation summarizes these challenges:

C'est qu'il y a un souci de … parce que c'est, c'est vrai. Parce que moi c'est, j'aurais pas eu le réflexe. C'est sûr qu'en pensant pendant deux minutes, oui c'est vrai. Mais j'avais, j'ai jamais pensé qu'il faudrait changer de condom, tu sais, avant de changer de partenaire, ça aussi tu sais ... Ce qui arrive avec un, un ... je sais pas moi, une soirée a six personnes par exemple ... C'est que tu vas pas penser a amener, il faut qu'il y ait au moins six condoms par, par gars ... C'est pas quelque chose a laquelle j'avais pensé au départ la ... C'est, c'est tout a fait logique, c'est juste que ... Étant donné que toute la, l'information est par rapport au euh ... a ça, c'est basé sur des échanges euh a deux personnes ... c'est pas le genre de détail que ... que j'avais entendu avant ça.

(It's that, there's an issue with, because, it's true. Me, I would not have thought of that. For sure, in thinking about it for two minutes, of course it's true. But I ... I had never thought that one had to change the condom, you know, before changing one's partner, that too, you know? What happens when, I don't know, an evening with six people for instance? It's that you're not going to think about bringing six condoms per man. It's not something I had thought about from the get-go. It's totally logical, it's just that, given that all the information is based on exchanges between two people, it's not the kind of detail I had ever heard about before.)

This man points out something that is, as he says, perhaps obvious but is not discussed in HIV prevention: education speaks of protected sexual relations between two individuals. Such an approach does not acknowledge the prevention issues at play in group sex – for instance, the necessity of using a new condom for each new sexual partner (or more accurately, for each new orifice). Such a practice is required in particular to avoid transmitting STDs. As one individual remarks,

La gaffe que le monde font, je disais, ils prennent un condom mettons pour deux femmes. Ça c'est plus bon ... Même si t'as un condom, t'es avec deux filles, s'il y en a une qui a quelque chose, ça va aller sur le condom pis tu vas le transmettre à l'autre ... Il faut que tu changes le condom. T'as pas le choix là.

(The error that people make, I was saying, they take a condom for two women. That's not good. Even if you have a condom, with the two ladies, if one of them has something, it will go on the condom and you will transmit it to the other. You have to change the condom. You don't have a choice.)

The absence of this kind of information within HIV education illustrates the ways in which there remains a great deal of work to be done in the field. Moreover, given the frequency of simultaneous multiple partners for some (although certainly not all) bisexuals and swingers, a virtual absence of such practical information in HIV and STD education illustrates the extent to which these people and communities have been ignored within public health. The identification of such an absence is, as we have argued, more than a simple matter of content. It speaks to the question of knowledge more generally – the manner in which our information about HIV/AIDS prevention is organized. The men and women interviewed in our study contend that the framework of knowledge currently in vogue within public health assumes sexual relations between two individuals, ignoring other realities. That such a narrow conception of sexuality persists within the field of HIV prevention more than thirty years into an epidemic speaks to the force this particular knowledge paradigm holds.

Using Plain Language to Get a Message Across

The content of HIV education campaigns, then, is not well adapted to the sexual practices of many bisexuals and swingers: the full range of their sexual partners is not represented, and basic information to protect themselves and their partners against HIV and STDs is unavailable. In addition to such limits in substantive content, our study respondents provided us with useful data on the specific language often used in public health education. Many of the people interviewed, for instance, contend that effective health education needs to use the language of everyday people. They underlined the manner in which so much HIV education relies upon a specialized vocabulary that is familiar to people working in public health, but that remains foreign and confusing to the average person. The importance of using plain language in HIV work was made clear through two specific examples within the course of our research. When we began conducting our interviews, we asked people to tell us about their information needs concerning HIV and other sexually transmitted infections (STIs). The initialism *STI* is a recent development in the field of public health, and one that seeks to more accurately name certain conditions like chlamydia and gonorrhoea as *infections* rather than *diseases*. While such an appellation is technically correct, it quickly became clear to us that people did not understand either this initialism (STIs) or its long form, sexually transmitted infections. In our initial interviews, we had to explain what this term and collocation meant – an indication that, at the level of research methods, the question was not clear. Since the goal of research is to obtain relevant information, we adapted our questionnaire accordingly and referred to *sexually transmitted diseases* and *STDs*, which were concepts and terms familiar to the participants in our study. In chapter 7, we will discuss in more depth our decision to use these terms in the educational materials that we produced. For now, the point to be taken is that in order to communicate effectively with our interview subjects, we needed to speak a language that they understood.

The importance of using plain language in work on HIV (whether of research, policy, education, or services) was cited as fundamental to developing effective education. Such a premise became immediately apparent when we showed our interviewees examples of previous educational posters, in particular an advertisement from the Assumptions campaign. This poster includes the text message, 'He would have told me if he was positive. He would have told me if he was negative. How do you know what you know?' (In French, the text uses the word *seropositive* and *seronegative*, as their short forms are not commonly used to indicate HIV serostatus usage within francophone contexts.) Significantly, few of our respondents understood the language in question:

C'est quoi la différence entre séropositif et séronégatif? ... je savais que séropositif ça veut dire que tu l'as. Mais séronégatif, je le savais pas ce que ça voulait dire.

(What's the difference between seropositive and seronegative? I knew that seropositive means that you have it. But seronegative, I didn't know what that meant.)

Il me l'aurait dit si, s'il était séro ... séropositif euh ... Je suis pas sûr de ça là. Tu sais.

(He would have told me if he was sero ... seropositive. I'm not sure about that. You know.)

The fact that this term represents an insider language familiar to those working in public health was underlined by several of our respondents:

Parce que peut-être que c'est comme ... peut-être que c'est un autre vocabulaire qui est comme fréquemment employé là, mais la séronégativité là ou les séronégatifs autour de moi là, c'est peut-être parce qu'il y a juste ça là, mais j'ai jamais employé ça, il y a jamais personne qui m'a dit « je suis séropositif », jamais.

(Because maybe it's like … maybe it's another vocabulary that is frequently used, but seronegativity or seropositivity around me, it's maybe just that, but I've never used that, never has someone said to me, 'I am seropositive,' never.)

Parce qu'on entend ben plus dire 'séropositif.' Mais séronégatif là … on n'entend pas séronégatif.

(Because we hear 'seropositive' much more often. But seronegative, we never hear seronegative.)

The lack of familiarity with technical terms like *STI* and *séropositif* created confusion for many of our participants. (Here, we remind the reader that our recruitment was done in mainstream venues and primarily outside of AIDS service organizations. In this regard, many of our participants did not use the language of public health and AIDS agencies.) As outlined in the quotations above, terms like *séropositif* were not frequently used or understood. In several instances during the interviews, participants actually understood the opposite of what was intended, associating a 'seronegative' status with someone who has HIV, for example. Such a situation illustrates the negative consequences of employing a specialized vocabulary unfamiliar to many people: education designed to help people make informed decisions, and adopt safe behaviours, actually causes confusion.

The solution to such a dilemma is quite simple, according to the people with whom we spoke. HIV education needs to ensure that it uses a popular language that is sure to be understood by all. On the above advertisement as part of the Assumptions campaign, one of our interviewees suggested an alternative translation to bring home this point:

Sauf que la phrase [« il me l'aurait dit s'il était séropositif »], moi je trouve que c'est une phrase … quand tu veux aller chercher des affaires, des affaires aussi intimes chez les gens, si tu prends des mots qui sont pas les mots des gens, à quelque part je trouve que tu te tires dans le pied, tsé. Moi j'aurais mis plus une phrase genre, « le sida c'est pas écrit dans le front ». Tsé, tsé, une expression populaire, tsé.

(Except that the phrase ['he would have told me if he was positive'], me I think that it's a phrase, when you want to get at things, things that are really intimate for people, if you don't use people's words, at some level I think you're shooting yourself in the foot, you know. I would have used a phrase more like, 'AIDS is not stamped on somebody's forehead.' You know, a common expression, you know.)

Here, the person recognizes the importance of using common, everyday expressions in order to send a message. While the specific translation proposed may in fact not be the most nuanced at the level of science and virology (it is the virus of HIV that can be transmitted, and not AIDS per se), this particular suggestion employs the idiomatic expressions of Québec language and society in order to reach a mainstream audience. Like a use of the term *STD*, the phrase proposed begins with the language and world view of ordinary folk. According to the people we interviewed, then, effective public health education needs to begin with a non-specialist vocabulary (see Massé 1995).

Diversity of People in Educational Campaigns: Age, Culture,
Multiple Sexual Partners, Beauty

Participants raised more general concerns about the diversity of people represented within HIV advertisements and campaigns. In addition to claiming the need to include women (more on this subject in the next chapter), they wanted to ensure that images included people of all ages:

R : Franchement là, il y en a pas beaucoup [d'annonces vih].
Q : Il y en a pas beaucoup?
R : Pour les hommes de mon âge là.

(R: I mean really, there aren't a lot [of HIV ads].
Q: There aren't a lot?
R: For men of my age.

Some participants raised issues that are specific to certain older women:

Pis tsé il y en a qui ont pas fait l'amour depuis dix ans, quinze ans, vingt ans, vingt-cinq ans, ils pensent que la première personne … ah ben là je suis sortie avec, c'est un bon monsieur là … on a pas besoin de ça, on a tous les deux été mariés longtemps, on a pas besoin de ça les condoms là.

(And you know there are those who haven't made love in ten, fifteen, twenty, twenty-five years, they think that the first person … oh well, I've gone out with him, he's a good man, we don't need that, we were both married a long time, we don't need those condoms.)

Moi je trouve ça … parce que les … ça regroupe, les personnes âgées aussi entre soixante ans, cinquante, mais âgées je dis entre cinquante et soixante-dix ans … Eux autres ils ont quasiment couché toute leur vie sans condom … Il y en a qui … leur femme, des fois il y en a comme euh qui décèdent. Fait qu'ils se retrouvent une nouvelle euh … ils se rencontrent une nouvelle femme, mais lui le monsieur ou la madame ont été habitués sans condom … Mais ça fait aussi que ça amène aussi des personnes âgées qui … qui tombent avec des IST ou juste des maladies transmissibles sexuellement … Eux autres sont pas assez euh … ils sont pas assez sensibilisés. Là aussi on les, on les a comme tassés … Parce que les personnes âgées on dit toujours qu'ils ont pas de sexualité … Ou on veut pas le savoir. Mais, ils en ont.

(Me, I find that, it includes older people in their sixties, fifties, older, but like between fifty and seventy years old. For them, they've had sex almost their entire lives without condoms. And some of them, sometimes some of their wives die. So they find a new one, they meet a new woman, but the man or the woman is not used to condoms. So you end up with older people too who have STIs or sexually transmitted diseases. They are not educated enough. There again, we've like tossed them aside. Because older people, it's always said, don't have a sexuality. We don't want to know about it. But they do.)

Still other interviewees contend that HIV education could confront the myth that with age comes responsibility:

Ben tu sais qu'on voit mettons euh … tu sais, un couple qui était … tu sais à mettons euh qui, tu sais un, je dis pas un vrai couple infecté là, mais supposément, mais qui sont, tu sais hors de ceux qu'on cible d'habitude genre. Comme exemple, on voit un couple, une petite Ginette avec un petit Yves genre là … Tu sais, qui ont l'air vraiment normal, straight là. Mais que tu sais, ils disent dedans mettons qu'ils sont échangistes pis qu'ils l'ont attrapé en faisant un échange genre. Parce qu'ils pensaient que des personnes responsables de leur âge peuvent pas avoir ça genre.

(Well you know when we see, you know, a couple, I mean not a real couple who has been infected, but supposedly so, but who are, you know, outside of who is normally targeted type of thing. For example, we see a couple, a little Ginette and a little Yves type. You know, they look really normal, really straight. But you know, they say there that they are swingers and they got it through swapping. Because they thought that responsible people of their age couldn't get that type of thing.)

The type of advertisement suggested above is one that seeks to remind the viewer that HIV can affect people of all ages and social backgrounds.

In addition to inclusion of different age groups, our interviewees maintain that HIV education in Québec needs to make more serious efforts in ethnocultural communities. For some people, this means including non-white people in campaign materials:

Écoute, comment développer des outils? Je pense que la première chose à faire c'est de garder en tête que tous les élèves ne sont pas blancs, catholiques, canadiens, québécois ... Je pense que c'est la première chose à garder en tête. Je pense qu'il faut développer des outils de plusieurs langues ... déjà l'anglais et français, c'est clair. Mais qu'ils soient parlant aussi à des communautés immigrantes ... Noire, arabe, asiatique ... haïtienne, martienne, je m'en fous.

(Listen, how to develop materials? I think the first thing to do is to keep in mind that not all the students are white, Catholic, Canadian, Québécois ... I think that's the first thing to keep in mind. I think you have to develop materials in several languages ... already French and English, that's clear. But that they also speak to immigrant communities ... black, Arab, Asian ... Haitian, Martian, I don't care.)

Il faut que tu prennes des gens noirs, blancs, asiatiques, euh je veux dire, ces campagnes-là tout le monde est blanc tout le temps, tsé ... Pourquoi? Les asiatiques ils baisent pas? Les femmes musulmanes, elles baisent elles aussi. Tsé, je veux dire c'est comme on cible tout le temps les mêmes gens pis on dirait qu'on oublie tous les gens différents autour.

(You have to use people who are black, white, Asian. I mean, those campaigns where all the people are always white, you know. Why? Asians

don't have sex? Muslim women, they have sex too. You know, I mean it's
like we're always targeting the same people and it's like we forget all the
other different people around.)

Yet inclusion of ethnocultural people and realities is more than a matter
of thinking about who is represented. For some participants, the general tone and approach of existing education is not necessarily adapted
to different ethnocultural realities within the city of Montréal. One
participant commented on the advertisement distributed in bars that
represented bed headboards in a cemetery with the caption, 'Le sida
tue encore' [AIDS still kills]:

> There's some differences in terms of how, you know, men relate to women,
> culturally speaking. You know? And I know a lot of people, like in the
> Asian community. And … like I'm from the West Indies, but you know, I
> know Jamaicans and stuff. And, I think, I don't know if it would help if the
> ads were … ah, you know, 'cause it's very … it's walking a fine line but,
> speaking to certain groups of people, but I don't know if … if … OK, for
> example a young eighteen-year-old Haitian guy would really be affected
> by this [reference to ad, 'AIDS still kills'].

Here, the question of 'inclusion' of different ethnocultural realities is figured not in exclusive relation to non-white bodies on a poster or in a pamphlet. Rather, the overall theme and tenor of a campaign is considered to
the extent that it would appeal to specific ethnocultural communities.

The question of diversity within prevention education, for respondents in our study, includes the varied realities of bisexuals such as
multiple partners. If, as we have seen, education does not contain
images or information adapted to the sexual practices of many people
who have sexual relations with both men and women, an appropriate
response is the development of educational materials that provide such
visuals and information:

> De rajouter du monde là. Pis sans que ce soit trop de gens là, mais de …
> parce que il y en a de plus en plus des trios, il y en a de plus en plus des,
> des couples qui sont avec d'autres couples.

> (Add some people there. Not that there would be too many people, but,
> maybe because there are more and more trios, more and more couples
> who are with other couples.)

Je suis pas, je suis pas scientifique pis je pense pas de l'être [inaudible] à tout là mais ... c'est ça, que je ferais peut-être une annonce comme euh ... je sais pas moi, « à trois, à quatre ou à plusieurs » ... « N'oubliez pas que la protection est toujours de mise ».

(I'm not ... I'm not a scientist but ... I would maybe create an ad with like, I don't know, 'three, four or more' ... 'Don't forget that protection is always necessary.')

But just recognizing the fact that people have multiple partners. I think that's something that I don't really see that much.

Ah mon dieu, oui, il y a un gros défi ... Le problème que j'ai rencontré souvent dans la, dans l'association, je dirais c'est le conjoint ou la conjointe qui est marié pis qui va voir ailleurs et qui se protège pas et qui revient à la maison, toujours pas protégé ... C'est que si tu switches de partenaire ou si t'as un, un comme on dit un, un partenaire stable mais que tu en as un autre qui est moins, euh, protège-toi. Tsé. Si t'as un partenaire pendant dix ans pis tu vas jamais ailleurs pendant dix ans parce que t'as pas l'attirance, ben la journée si tu y vas, protège-toi.

(Oh my God, that's a big challenge. The problem that I've run into often, in the association, I would say is when the partner who is married and who goes to get some on the side and does not protect themselves and comes back home, still unprotected. It's that if you change partners or if you have a, like we say, a stable partner but you have one who is less so, well protect yourself. If you have a partner for ten years and you never go elsewhere for ten years because you have attraction, well the day that you do go, protect yourself.)

Je sais pas comment ils pourraient mettre un concept où est-ce que il y a ... c'est bisexuel sans faire un threesome genre là. Fait que c'est comme ... s'ils étaient capables de le faire sans que ça l'air de ça, parce que souvent le monde ils pensent ça aussi, tsé.

(I don't know how they could put such a concept in place where it's like bisexual, without making a threesome. It's like that ... if they were able to do that without it being, because often people think it's like that, you know.)

In related ways, all of these quotations underline the importance of recognizing the fact of multiple partners when speaking about sexuality, whether that be a partner outside of a primarily monogamous relationship, sexual relations with both men and women, or group sex with a number of different partners simultaneously. Our participants contend that attention to diversity within HIV prevention needs to represent a variety of sexualities and sexual practices, including multiple partners.

One final issue addressed in the content of existing sexual health education is the physical beauty of the people in most campaigns. Our interviewees contend that most of the education they see only has images of 'beautiful' people, in a manner similar to other marketing strategies.

> Q : Alors vous vous reconnaissez dans la publicité?
> R : Ben pas nécessairement dans le genre, ça dépend laquelle là, des genres de ... je me reconnais dans le sens de personnes qui ont des relations ... Mais pas physiquement, je me reconnais pas. C'est ça que je veux dire.

> (Q: So do you see yourself in the publicity?
> R: Well not necessarily in that type, it depends on which type, which types ... I see myself in the sense of people who have relations ... But not physically, I don't see myself. That's what I'm saying.)

> Souvent aussi quand on voit dans les magazines gais, j'aime pas les stéréotypes. Le, le bel homme musclé euh ... pas de poil, tout plein d'huile là ... J'ai beaucoup de difficulté avec ces stéréotypes là. Les gais magnifiques là ... ça pour moi ça m ... ça m'atteint pas, ça me touche pas.

> (Often when one sees gay magazines, I don't like stereotypes. The beautiful muscled man ... no hair, all oiled. I have a lot of difficulty with those stereotypes. The magnificent gays, that for me, that doesn't reach me, that doesn't do anything for me.)

Promotional materials that rely on cultural stereotypes of physical beauty alienate many of the people we interviewed. As the last quotation makes clear, this is especially notable for men who may have sexual relations with other men, but who do not participate actively in gay life and its symbols, iconography, and standards of physical beauty. The development of prevention materials that include pictures of ordinary, everyday people was cited as a necessary strategy for more effective HIV education.

Our research has revealed that there are important limits to the content of current HIV prevention materials, especially diversity. In most campaigns there is an absence of women, people from ethnocultural communities, individuals of different age ranges, people who have multiple sexual partners, and people with different kinds of bodies and physical beauty. Such absences constitute important limits to reaching a wide variety of people, notably individuals who have sexual relations with both men and women.

The Need for Practical Information

More than simply criticizing gaps in educational materials, our interviewees provided useful, pro-active suggestions about the kind of content needed in prevention materials. The inclusion of concrete, practical information was cited as especially important in this regard. For many people interviewed, HIV education remains general and vague, with simple messages to 'use a condom' or 'protect yourself.' This kind of approach does not offer people the information they need, aside from an encouragement to use condoms for penetrative sexual relations. The following quotations bring these issues to light. Reacting to the 'AIDS still kills' campaign distributed in bars, respondents underline how this advertisement does not offer people a way to act on knowledge:

A lot went into this. For what? Is there anything you've learned about AIDS, HIV, or how to protect yourself, how to protect your friends? Anything in that? No. Have you learned anything? Not one thing.

Hmmm, that's nice. But there's not much prevention it's just stating that ... HIV kills ... We all know that ... that we all know, but again there's no prevention, I mean ... There's not even a site where we could click on, like ... like no information where to get information to protect.

Le sida tue encore. Bon, c'est ça. Il y a pas de prévention là-dedans là ... En tous cas, moi je vois pas ça comme une prévention là.

(AIDS still kills. OK, that's it. There is no prevention within that. In any case, I don't see that as prevention.)

This sentiment was echoed in other interviews in discussing education on STDs:

Ils disaient juste : « Bon, euh telle situation c'est à risque, vous pouvez attraper telle maladie » ... « Voici les symptômes, à quoi ça se ressemble ». Mais ils disaient pas comment on peut éviter cette situation là. Ça a été comme ma seule déception là ... C'était plus de l'information sur c'est quoi telle MTS ou telle ITS. Bon euh ... plutôt que comment l'éviter là.

(They just said, 'Well, this situation is risky, you could get a disease.' 'Here are the symptoms, what they look like.' But they didn't say how you can avoid this situation. That was my only disappointment. It was more information about what such-and-such an STD or STI is, rather than how to avoid it.)

The consequences of a general approach to HIV prevention could be serious, in that the information offered does not help people in their actions. At times, a vague message of HIV prevention such as 'wear a condom' could actually have negative unintended consequences, including *increasing* the likelihood of transmitting STDs. The person interviewed below outlines how this is especially relevant within a context of group sexual relations:

Il y a ben du monde qui, qui font comme, « Ah j'ai un condom ». Ouais, mais regarde, si tu changes de femmes pareil là ... C'est beau se protéger, mais il faut que tu penses aux autres aussi dans un sens là ... t'as pas le choix ... Il faut pas que tu penses juste à ta propre personne ... Ben oui, j'ai jamais vu quelque chose là-dessus pour le vrai ... Le monde disent, « Oui mais je porte un condom ». Oui mais regarde, il faut que tu le changes ton condom [*rires*]. T'as pas le choix.

(There are lots of people, who are like, 'Well I have a condom.' Yes well, look, if you change female partners, just the same ... It's good to protect yourself, but in a sense you also have to think about others. You don't have a choice. You can't just think about yourself. So yeah, I've never seen something on that for real. People say, 'Yes but I am wearing a condom.' Yes well look, you have to change your condom [*laughs*]. You don't have a choice.)

This quotation underlines the need for educational materials that give people the practical information they require to make informed decisions – such as changing a condom for each new partner. Without such a practical approach, HIV education remains at a vague level, and people mistakenly believe that they are responsible in protecting themselves and others against all kinds of STDs.

Careful attention to the voices of the men and women interviewed reveals that they have identified specific information needs with regards to HIV/AIDS, but to STDs as well. Indeed, the importance of addressing sexual health broadly was underlined in our interviews:

> qu'il y a pas euh d'autre, assez de ... tu sais le, le sida, le VIH euh ... euh même l'hépatite il y a beau ... beaucoup. Mais les autres euh sont un peu euh ... laissés tu sais.

> (that there are not other, you know, AIDS, HIV, even hepatitis, there are many. But the others are a little bit ... neglected, you know.)

> Mais c'est parce que il y a pas juste euh le VIH là ... Pis ça devrait pas être séparé des ... des MTS tant qu'à moi.

> (But it's because there isn't just HIV. And that shouldn't be separated from other STDs, in my opinion.)

In keeping with a need for practical information, people articulated a desire to have education on both STDs and HIV. Since they are all part of general sexual health, it is appropriate for education to address them comprehensively.

Linking STD and HIV information is part of a broader approach to ensure that education begins with constructive, practical information:

> Condoms are not 100 per cent. So breaking down those simple answers for people with things like practical advice and alternatives in case of emergency. You know, things like that.

> People are scared to talk about sex. Even though they're talking about HIV prevention, they need to talk about things like what if I have a blister, or I just bit my tongue and I'm about to go down on my boyfriend or my girlfriend, can I lick their butt, balls? Sorry ... Chapped lips? What if we're getting too sweaty, scratches, does she have her period? This is what people need to know about. And I can't find anything ... Enough of beautiful full-colour brochures saying, 'Practise safe sex,' 'Put on a condom.' That's so not good enough, it's not even funny.

I think instead of telling you, 'You can die and you can die and you can die,' you could be like ... 'If you die, well this is how you stop it.' ... Chop it up a little bit with ... not just criticisms but proactives ... like constructive criticism ... OK, this is what you shouldn't do ... but this is what you should do. Not this shouldn't, shouldn't, shouldn't, shouldn't, shouldn't.

The challenge for meaningful prevention, according to these voices, is to begin proactively and to suggest concrete things that people can do in their sexual lives to protect themselves and their partners from HIV and STDs. While such an approach may seem obvious, it is striking nonetheless that it is relatively rare in HIV education. The analysis provided by one participant in particular – who exposes the ways in which a message of 'Wear a condom' does not address the complexities of group sex – offers particular insight into how general messages devoid of practical information can have disastrous consequences, putting women in particular at risk for STDs. Here, the woman interviewed makes an important critique of how our knowledge of HIV and STD prevention is structured, a framework that ignores group sexual practices and the specific vulnerabilities of women to HIV and STD. This kind of research result, then, suggests that we need to organize our knowledge of HIV education differently.

Suggested Formats for HIV Education

In addition to requesting substantive content, participants offer suggestions about different ways HIV education could be packaged, formatted, and delivered. The suggestions provide a wide range of options and possibilities, ranging from the more traditional posters and pamphlets to somewhat more innovative ideas, such as a hot air balloon in the form of a condom! Suggestions included tactics specific to the Internet (Internet advertisements, pop-up windows on relevant sites), educational trailers shown in the cinema, booklets developed specifically for swingers, interactive games and activities marketed specifically to youth, advertisements on banners flown behind a plane, classified advertisements, bookmarks, radio advertisements, refrigerator magnets, and information contained in a 'Publi-sac' – a bag of promotional flyers delivered free to Montréal homes weekly. Some suggestions reflect the specific context of a milieu. For example, one participant recounts how a swinger sauna has a system with signs on the door handle indicating the desired partner, such as 'Couple seeks couple' or 'Couple seeks single woman.' Integration of HIV and STD prevention messages within such signs would be an effective manner to promote sexual health within this milieu.

Participants claimed the need for a broad-based, mainstream campaign in order to reach people who have sexual relations with both men and women. An example of a famous billboard advertisement with a popular Québec singer, Marie-Chantal Toupin, was cited for its impact:

> Voyons, Marie-Chantal Toupin qui avait mis son affiche 'Regardez-moi dans les yeux' avec ses grosses boules sur le Pont Champlain, je mettrais une affiche comme ça juste pour faire justement encore sacrer le monde dans leur auto, qu'ils disent tabernouche là, mais ils l'ont vue, ils vont s'en rappeler. Je ferais des choses choc comme ça au lieu justement montrer la beauté de la femme ou ces choses-là, je ferais des choses comme ça à la place qui ... Marie-Chantal, son affiche est restée là trois jours, mais le monde en parle encore, mais pourquoi qu'on ferait pas ça avec des publicités pour le sida ou des choses comme ça, que plusieurs années plus tard les gens se rappellent, ce qui veut dire qu'ils ont appris là-dedans.

> (Listen, Marie-Chantal Toupin, who put her poster 'Look me in the eyes' with her huge knockers on the Champlain bridge, I would put a poster up like that, precisely to annoy the people in their cars, so they say, 'Shit,' but they've seen it, they're going to remember it. I would do some shock things like that precisely to show the beauty of women or those kinds of things. I would do things like that as opposed to ... Marie-Chantal, her poster stayed up there three days, but people are still talking about it. Well, why don't we do that with AIDS ads or things like that, so that years later people remember, which means that they've learned from them?)

In keeping with the expressed need for practical information, one participant suggested an educational tool that summarizes the transmission, symptoms, incubation period, and treatment of different STDs:

> Tout le monde, dans toutes les maisons, devraient avoir un tableau de ça. Devraient avoir un tableau compact des MTS, des, des manières de transmission, avec qui, homme, femme, incubation. C'est comme compact, que tu garderais tsé comme ... Tout le monde devrait avoir ça ... ça devrait pas être à l'hôpital ou au CLSC ou ... Tsé. On est capable de garder des grosses

épaisseurs de dictionnaire mais on n'est pas capable de garder une feuille sur les maladies [transmissibles sexuellement].

(Everybody, in every house, should have a table of that. Should have a small table of STDs, the modes of transmission, with whom, man, woman, incubation. It's like small, that you could keep, you know … Everyone should have that. It shouldn't be at the hospital or the CLSC. We're able to keep big thick dictionaries but we're not able to keep a sheet on [sexually transmitted] diseases.)

Finally, interviewees maintain that education can also be provided when questions of HIV and STDs are incorporated within popular culture:

Tsé comme j'écoutais l'émission *Watatatow*, ils en ont un personnage qui a le sida là présentement pis je trouve ça super brillant qu'ils aient fait ça justement pour montrer regarde là, elle était pas à l'abri pis.

(You know, like I was watching the television show *Watatatow*, right now they have a character who has AIDS, and I find that really brilliant that they did that precisely to show that, look, she wasn't immune to it.)

Virginie le monde crie contre ça. C'est quand même … je trouve qu'elle passe quand même l'information que les gens osent pas poser … passer ailleurs.

(*Virginie* people shout against that. But even so … I find that they put out information that people would not dare pass around elsewhere.)

The formats suggested by participants, then, offer different ways to organize HIV prevention messages. Some of these formats are familiar, while others represent truly innovative strategies to get a message out into the public domain.

Conclusion

The data presented in this chapter bring to light some of the main weaknesses of current HIV and STD educational campaigns, particularly in reaching individuals who have sexual relations with both men and women. Regrettably, current HIV prevention neglects the diversity and full spectrum of people's sexual lives, as, for example, when campaigns address only the male partners of men who are sexually active with both men and women. The participants cited here have identified compelling problems with the content of most HIV education: a fear-based approach that alienates the viewer/reader; materials that are not adapted to the sexual lives of bisexuals and swingers (ignoring both male and female partners, as well as specific protection issues raised in a context of group sex); a technical and specialized vocabulary unfamiliar to everyday people; little attention to diversity in gender, culture, age, and physical beauty; and an absence of practical information to help people adopt safe sexual behaviours. Having outlined these gaps in prevention information, participants make suggestions that would significantly alter the kinds of information available in HIV education.

The participants cited throughout this chapter are often pragmatic. They provide concrete examples of the problems they find, as well as what could be done to make HIV information more relevant. Yet such a pragmatic component does not mean that these experiences are inapplicable to institutions. Indeed, the viewpoints in this chapter demonstrate insightful analysis of how knowledge is organized in and through institutions, as well as the way that legitimizing only certain forms of knowledge excludes people from the social world. In concluding this chapter, we examine these questions of knowledge in more depth here. The reliance on a technical language in HIV education provides a useful point of departure to explore these issues.

The concerns articulated about the use of a specialized vocabulary in HIV campaigns indicate that public health often works with its own insider language. Terms such as *STI, seropositive,* and *seronegative* are used commonly within public health settings, as well as within community-based AIDS organizations. Yet the participants in our study were unfamiliar with such language and were often confused about the specific meaning and intention of educational materials that rely upon such a specialized vocabulary. Public health education reflects a specific language, culture, and world view – one not necessarily shared by ordinary people. The way that it speaks about disease, disease prevention, and health promotion appeals to a certain way of understanding and naming the world. Such an understanding is shared by many AIDS service organizations as well, in that they work within such a context. Such detailed attention to the kind of language used in HIV education confirms one of the ideas advanced in chapter 2, that the work of HIV prevention is carried out by specific agencies deemed to have the appropriate expertise in this area. The distribution of a large-scale, national educational campaign (such as the Assumptions campaign described above) assumed that the reader/viewer would understand a health promotion message organized around the terms *seropositive* and *seronegative*. While that claim may or may not be true for gay men,[3] our research clearly demonstrates that this campaign caused confusion among bisexual men and women because they did not understand the language employed.

The use of technical vocabulary, common within many AIDS groups, confirms that the main actors and stakeholders in HIV education reflect a particular community of state-funded AIDS organizations. The use of a specialized AIDS language in HIV education, in other words, illustrates the extent to which the work is carried out by people considered to be experts in the field. The data presented here suggest that this is, in fact, a weakness: this type of education excludes different, more common ways of knowing about HIV and ensures that only the usual suspects are recognized to have expertise in the field. The use of a technical vocabulary in HIV education, then, illustrates the ways in which the development of HIV educational materials is circular, involving representatives of certain AIDS agencies recognized and funded by the state. The voices in this chapter highlight a radically different interpretation of information and bring to light the disjuncture between their information needs and those offered within HIV education. This dynamic embodies a 'line of fault' explored in greater depth in chapter 2. People who have sexual relations with both men and women have needs for HIV information that is different from the knowledge offered by public health and community-based HIV/AIDS organizations. By speaking directly with such individuals, we can better understand how HIV/AIDS institutions function, as well as the ways in which these agencies exclude certain realities and people.

The next chapter continues to explore this problematic, with specific attention to questions of gender in HIV and STD educational campaigns.

5 'Cherchez la femme': The Exclusion of Women in HIV Education and Services

But I still feel like it's targeted towards gay men mostly. Or young gay men. I don't know if I've ever seen an AIDS-specific ad that was heterosexual at all.
– Study participant

As we have seen in previous chapters, the work of institutions is carried out by individuals who bring their own knowledge, biases, and interests to the work they do. We illustrated this point with a discussion of community-based AIDS organizations who argued that our work was not community-based, because it was not taking place in state-funded sites of AIDS education and services. Here, the perspective of some individuals on how we define 'community' shaped the workings of a grant program. Additional feedback on our application for funds to conduct this research project sheds light on the social relations of HIV / AIDS work in Canada and Québec. The comment can be considered curious, outrageous, or deeply instructive. The grant program funded community-based HIV / AIDS research, and the element under consideration was the expertise of the research team. Did we as applicants provide enough information, in other words, to demonstrate that we had the relevant academic background and community engagement to conduct the proposed research? One evaluator maintained that the research team proposed was competent, 'although very feminist, which risks creating bias vis-à-vis the research to be undertaken.'[1] We should emphasize here that this was not necessarily the opinion of the entire evaluation committee, but merely that of one member.[2] Nonetheless, the comment does raise a host of questions, perhaps especially because the feedback did not contain clarify why it was a bad thing to be 'too feminist' in research about sexual health. Indeed, to contend in 2004 that one can be 'very feminist' in HIV/AIDS research argues that some feminist scholars and activists have gone too far in their approach and political demands. It is to suggest that one can be too critical in an attention to questions of gender in research and education related to HIV/AIDS. Indeed, the reviewer states outright that if one goes too far in feminist analysis within HIV/AIDS, one is producing knowledge that is biased, partisan, or even harmful.

We bring this anecdote to light because it reveals the unease that at least one evaluator experiences with feminist research. (We note here, as well, that the feedback offered is an objection to a feminist approach to research, and much less to the expertise of our research team – feminist or otherwise.) A comment that one can be 'very feminist' in HIV/AIDS research is instructive, because it illustrates the extent to which the importance of attending to women's issues is still an argument that has to be made within HIV/AIDS funding. In the absence of a generalized understanding of this question, the biases of individual review committee members will continue to create barriers to funding research projects that clearly integrate women's realities.

The substance of this comment, while perhaps alarming from a feminist perspective, is alas not surprising for many of us working in the field of HIV/AIDS. As we have seen, in its early days clinical definitions of AIDS did not consider the specific effects of HIV in women's bodies, such that women were excluded from many official AIDS diagnoses (ACT-UP/NY 1990; Epstein 1996; Gorna 1996). At a more grassroots, community-based level, one can also observe the emergence of specific organizations dedicated to women and HIV: in Canada, one can cite Voices of Positive Women in Toronto, or le Centre de ressources et d'interventions en santé et sexualité (now defunct) and the Comité Sida Montréal – Femmes in Montréal. These agencies emerged in part because women were not able to access the kind of information or services they required within mainstream HIV/AIDS agencies. Particularly at a community level, the development and emergence of women's HIV/AIDS organizations occurred in some instances through profound struggle and frustration. Women expressed anger that their specific issues were not being considered, let alone addressed, within organizations that had been established by men (ACT-UP/NY; Epstein; Gorna). In certain cases, women branched off to form their own sites to create education and services, because they did not feel they could work well within the existing network of agencies. This is not to say that, historically, all AIDS service organizations were hostile to women, but it is to underline that an ignorance of women's issues characterized the early years of the epidemic and that feminist health advocates in HIV/AIDS organized themselves accordingly. The comment that our research team risks creating biased knowledge, then, is bound within an institutional location of HIV/AIDS research and organizations that have not always served women well. This particular evaluative comment reminds us of the extent to which HIV/AIDS research and services remain insensitive to women's issues.

If citing this comment allows us to understand more clearly the invisible workings of gender in the institutional work of funding HIV/AIDS research and services, for the purposes of the present study, we must also ask the necessary corollary question: do everyday women feel that they have access to the HIV/AIDS information they require? This chapter considers this question in depth. Drawing on women's voices, we examine the ways in which HIV campaigns in Québec are implicitly gendered. The women we interviewed argue that women's bodies, lives, and experiences are frequently – sometimes consistently – absent from HIV/AIDS education.

Cherchez la femme

For some participants, a lack of consideration of women's issues reflects a more general absence of mainstream HIV education:

> Mais c'est sûr que il, il y a pas de campagne. C'est pas qu'il y en a pas assez, c'est qu'il y en a pas, tout simplement. J'en vois pas.

> (But it's obvious there are no campaigns. It's not that there aren't enough, it's that there aren't any, quite simply. I don't see any.)

> R : Il y en a moins qu'avant … Euh il y en a pu beaucoup.
> Q : Et comment vous expliquez ça?
> R : Euh peut-être que ils ont vu que c'était comme une sorte de mode. D'après moi c'est ça. Parce que ils en parlent pu pantoute.

> (R: There are fewer than before. There aren't many at all now.
> Q: And how would you explain that?
> R: Well, maybe they saw it as a sort of fashion. To me, it's that. Because they don't talk about it at all anymore.)

Il y a un gros laisser aller. Il y a pas assez de ... il y a rien qui accroche. Ils font ben plus pour la crisse de cigarette.

(There's a tremendous lack of action. There aren't enough, nothing grabs your attention. They do more for those damn cigarettes.)

Some participants contend that while there are certain campaigns in Québec, these generally target gay male communities.

But I still feel like it's pretty targeted towards gay men mostly. Or young gay men. I don't know if I've ever seen an AIDS-specific ad that was heterosexual at all.

If the only education available is directed to gay men, then women are excluded from prevention initiatives.[3] Interviewees also had the impression that since most information was concentrated in the gay village (a specific neighbourhood in Montréal), campaigns were invisible outside of this location:

Je vois pas grande chose. Quand je suis pas au centre-ville, je vois rien de ça. C'est ça qui arrive, il y en a pas partout là. Tu sais, ils devraient en mettre partout des pancartes pis des affaires là. Je le sais pas ... tu sais comme moi je suis à Saint-Léonard. À St-Léonard, ils en parlent pas. T'en ... t'entendras pas parler de ça ben ben.

(I haven't really seen anything. When I'm not downtown, I don't see any of that. That's what happens, they don't have it everywhere. You know, they should put posters and billboards up everywhere. I don't know, you know, like me, I'm in Saint-Léonard. In St-Léonard, nobody talks about it. You won't really hear anything about that.)

Je trouve que c'est beaucoup centré là dans une partie euh de la ville. Euh ... si tu vas à, dans l'est ... il y a à chaque coin de rue un, un, un ressource de ça [la toxicomanie]. Mais tu vas à l'Ouest euh ... qui, il y a rien, absolument rien. Tu sais.

(I find it's really concentrated in a certain part of the city. If you go east, on every corner there's an organization [that deals with drug use]. But if you go west there's absolutely nothing. You know.)

Je pense surtout pour des femmes. Je pense qu'il y a beaucoup de l'information qui est là, mon impression c'est que c'est plutôt pour les hommes ... Les seules choses que je vois c'est dans le village gai pis c'est toujours avec des photos des hommes.

(I'm thinking especially about women. I think there's a lot of information that's there, my impression is that it's really for men. The only things that I see are in the gay village and it's always photos of men.)

While these quotations highlight the spatial distribution of HIV education within the city, there is a gendered dimension to this dynamic. They underline that they see HIV education only in the gay village – a location in which the specific content speaks only about men's bodies. Thus, to argue that HIV education is not widely available across the island of Montréal is also to contend that campaigns have not addressed women in any systemic or targeted manner.

A few interviewees cited the visibility of campaigns directed to heterosexuals, as well as those targeting gay men. However, they noted that there was an absence of information that was specific to lesbian or bisexual women:

Like, I feel it's really specific to gay men, or really specific to straight couples or straight people. I don't remember seeing anything that's dyke- or bisexual-oriented. And I think that there are some specific things about being bi or being lesbian that aren't represented in that kind of media or whatever.

Un nouveau sauna que ça fait pas longtemps qu'il est ouvert, c'est un sauna mixte ... Il y a des hommes et des femmes. Euh là j'ai vu des panneaux publicitaires euh pour hommes. J'en n'ai pas vu pour femmes par contre.

(A new sauna that hasn't been open for long, it's a mixed sauna. There are men and women. And I've seen prevention posters for men. But I haven't seen anything for women.)

The gaps in information available to women was contrasted with that available to men:

J'ai remarqué que au niveau de la prévention des MTS l'information pour les relations sexuelles justement là euh ... je va appeler ça « homoféminines » donc … les relations entre femmes … que c'est pas du tout traité. Il y a une absence totale d'information sur la prévention des MTS … Par contre, du côté homosexuel masculin, ils ont toute la gamme d'informations euh … sur la prévention, les MTS, etc.

(I've noticed that, in terms of STD prevention education for sexual relations, precisely, I'll call them 'homo-feminine,' the relations between women, they are not dealt with at all. There is a complete absence of information on STD prevention. On the other hand, on the side of male homosexuals, they have the whole gamut of information, prevention, STDs, etc.)

As this observation makes clear, public health education on homosexualities is gendered, offering information and services to men and neglecting women entirely.

The data we gathered in our study include a critique of the manner in which campaigns seldom include women as sexual subjects, concentrating on the male partners of men who have sexual relations with both men and women. In a consideration of the Assumptions advertisement, one participant explains the manner in which this poster excludes women:

Ben c'est plus une annonce qui est pour les gais … Tsé, 'Il me l'aurait dit s'il était séropositif.' C'est pas du tout focussé pour une femme … C'est vraiment focussé pour les hommes … Pour euh l'homosexualité … C'est très bien focussé, c'est très bien ciblé … Tsé. Mais c'est pas ciblé pour la bisexuelle … Tu vas le focusser pour un homme bisexuel. Mais pas avec son approche avec la femme. Ça l'éduquera pas sur son ap, sur sa, son approche avec la femme.

(Well it's an ad that's more for gays. You know, 'He would have told me if he was positive.' It's not at all focused on a woman. It's really focused on men. For homosexuality. It's really well focused, well targeted. But it's not targeted to a bisexual woman. You're going to focus on a bisexual man. But not in terms of his approach with a woman. Because it won't educate him on his relations with a woman.)

This quotation examines the ways in which HIV education directed to men who have sex with men ignores the female partners of such men. It shows how the kind of HIV education that is currently available is also gendered, to the extent that women are absent. This is a critique centrally concerned with the knowledge we have of HIV education – especially in the context of 'MSM' populations – and it illustrates the ways in which our understanding of this disease is androcentric.

In their interviews, some of the respondents raised an argument that is sometimes used to justify the lack of HIV education specific to bisexuality. Within this discourse, it is contended that even though there may not be campaigns specific to bisexuals, people with bisexual behaviour can access the information they need by referring to both mainstream, heterosexual campaigns and initiatives addressing same-sex relations. Indeed, in meetings with public health officials, researchers, doctors, and service providers we were often confronted with such an argument. People questioned the relevance of our research with the contention that the information was already available, albeit perhaps not in the best form. One study participant addresses this argument up front and analyses how it makes certain assumptions about the sex and gender of people targeted for HIV prevention:

> R : Parce que souvent j'ai entendu dire euh, « oui, un peu euh que les bi peuvent euh piocher dans les campagnes hétéros » … « et piocher dans les campagnes homos et pis ils vont.» Ils en font leur euh … à leur tête euh …
> Q : Qu'est-ce que t'en penses de ça? Est-ce que …
> R : Jusqu'à un certain point. Mais euh … j'appliquerais beaucoup plus ça aux, aux hommes bisexuels … Là à ce moment là, oui ils peuvent piocher des deux côtés … Mais comme je disais tantôt, pour moi qui suis femme, c'est une autre paire de manches. Oui, je peux piocher du côté des campagnes hétérosexuelles pour la prévention euh … des MTS quand je suis avec un homme. Mais avec une femme … où sont les campagnes? Voilà. C'est là tout le problème. Donc, je peux pas piocher nulle part. Parce que ça, c'est pas du tout traité.

> (R: Because I've often heard, 'Well the bi's can get information from hetero campaigns' … 'and from gay campaigns,' and they will … they'll make sense of it themselves.
> Q: And what do you think about that? Is that …
> R: Up to a point. But I would apply that much more to bisexual men. At this time, yes they can get information from both sides. But like I said earlier, for me as a woman, it's another kettle of fish. Yes, I can get prevention information from heterosexual campaigns, STDs for when I am with a man. But with a woman … where are the campaigns? There you

have it. That's the real problem. So I can't get information anywhere. Because it's not dealt with at all.)

This woman offers an astute analysis of the individual who is so often assumed to be receiving HIV information. The argument that bisexuals can simply consult information developed for heterosexuals and homosexuals assumes that the bisexuals in question are men, since there are no campaigns that address woman-to-woman transmission of HIV and other STDs.

The lack of information on STDs and HIV transmission between women was further explained by our interviewees:

> Mais encore une fois j'ai l'impression que si ils font une campagne publicitaire ou ils donnent l'information sur la bisexualité, ils vont plus axer sur ... entre hommes disons, tsé, parce qu'on dirait que les gens pensent qu'entre femmes c'est immunisé, qu'il n'y a pas de danger.

> (But once again, I have the impression that if they do a campaign or give information about bisexuality, there going to focus more on ... between men, let's say, because it's as if people think that between women there is no risk.)

More than simply noting the absence of women in prevention materials, this woman critically analyses the causal relations underlying such a gap. The idea that women who have sexual relations with other women are not at risk for HIV and STDs justifies the lack of information campaigns addressing this matter. As we argue in chapter 1, mainstream epidemiology in public health frequently underestimates the vulnerability of woman-to-woman transmission of HIV and STDs (Bauer and Welles 2001). Researchers and policymakers then appeal to such distorted data to state that there is no specific need for a woman-to-woman HIV and STD prevention campaign. The women in our study explain the ways in which the minimization of risk between women informs a lack of action in this area:

> Ben je pense que les filles euh bisexuelles ont plus tendance à faire attention avec les gars pis beaucoup moins avec les filles ... Tsé je pense que souvent les filles partent avec l'idée que ... tu peux moins attraper des trucs entre filles, tsé ... Mais je sais que tu peux très bien attraper des trucs

entre filles … Pis on a tendance à plus se faire confiance entre filles, ce qui est un peu niaiseux finalement, tsé.

(Well I think that bisexual women have a tendency to pay attention when they are with men, and much less so with women … You know, often I think that the girls have the idea that … that you can't catch things between women. But I know that you can catch things between women. And we have this tendency to trust each other between women, which in the end is a bit silly, you know.)

The men and women we interviewed, then, provide both documentation of the absence of women in existing education and causal analysis of how this situation has been produced. Importantly, they go on to underline the importance of information that is both relevant and adapted to their lives, since they need such information in order to inform their actions:

My friends, there's two women, one is HIV-positive, one is not. They came to me to look for specific answers. They just couldn't find answers to these really specific questions that are crucial, critical. That's what they need to know to know how to behave and conduct themselves.

This quotation is instructive for a number of reasons. In the first instance, it highlights the difficulties women experience in finding relevant information – the women in question approached a male friend for information about HIV because they could not find appropriate information elsewhere. Second, the question of woman-to-woman transmission of HIV and STDs is far from abstract if it is known that one partner in a couple is HIV-positive. Indeed, the importance of having accurate information in order to adopt safe sexual behaviour was signalled by our interviewees:

Je veux dire, j'ai déjà connu euh … une fille qui avait une blonde. Et euh elle avait attrapé euh justement là l'herpes. Elle était toute surprise euh … J'ai dit, « Mais comment tu peux avoir attrapé l'herpès [*ricane*], tu sais » … Pis sa première réponse c'est, « Ben … comment veux-tu que je prévienne ça? Je le sais même pas comment m'y prendre ». Pis moi je me grattais la tête pis j'ai dit, « Mais … à bien y penser, moi non plus je ne le saurais pas quoi faire à ta place ».

(I mean, I know a woman who had a girlfriend. And she got herpes. She was all surprised. I said, 'Well, how could you have gotten herpes?' [*laughter*] You know. And her first reaction was, 'Well, how am I supposed to prevent that? I don't even know where to begin.' And I scratched my head and said, 'Well, having really thought about it, I wouldn't know what to do in your place either.')

The realities addressed in this citation, in which a woman is infected with herpes when she is with a female partner, belie the importance of providing accurate information. While the transmission of infections among women may occur less frequently than among men (although we remind the reader here that we do not have accurate data in this regard), transmission occurs nonetheless, and bisexual women in particular indicate higher rates of both HIV and STD prevalence than either lesbians or heterosexual women. Moreover, even if such a risk is considered to be 'less' than a parallel risk among men, the reality of the situation demands that people have the information they need to protect themselves. Our data suggest that women who have sexual relations with other women do not know the risk of transmitting HIV and STDs among women, to say nothing of what they can do concretely to prevent such transmission.

Indeed, the data from our interviews confirm the tremendous lack of information about woman-to-woman transmission of HIV and STDs. The people we spoke with had more questions than answers in this regard:

Q : Euh, est-ce que t'as des questions spécifiques concernant justement le VIH ou les infections transmises sexuellement?

R : Euh, j'en ai, j'en … euh, comme je, je suis vraiment pu à date là-dedans, pis d'ailleurs je pense que je suis devenue ignorante ou je ne sais quoi [*rires*]. Euh … tout ce qui est euh, quand on fait l'amour oral, je pense et je suis plus sûre, qu'on peut attraper des maladies là aussi. Mais quelles sont ces maladies-là, j'avoue que je suis perdue.

(Q: Do you have any specific questions concerning HIV or sexually transmitted infections?

R: I do, like, I'm not really up to date anymore. I think I've become ignorant or something (*laughs*). Everything about, um, when you have oral sex, I think but I'm not sure anymore, that you can get diseases there as well. What are those diseases, I confess I'm lost.)

I think I've got really inconsistent answers on [HIV transmission between] women ... on lesbians ... or ... sexual practices that are or are not risky ... My doctor is one of the people that ... that said something that [was] inconsist[ent] ... Just really inconsistent ... things about risk ... and practices I guess. And you don't, you just don't ... I guess ... safe sex with women was not an issue for me until I almost ... I was with a partner who told me after the fact, lied to me that she had herpes. Luckily I was unaffected but that really shocked me, and I guess since then I've taken it a lot more seriously, safe sex with women ... But before that, not at all. Not at all.

Q : Est-ce que tu as des questions en particulier concernant la prévention du VIH ou des infections sexuellement, est-ce qu'il y a ... ?

R : C'est ça que je me demandais si il y a un risque vrai ... mais je crois pas qu'il y a un risque très élévé dans la bisexualité entre femmes, en tout cas moins j'imagine que dans une relation hétérosexuelle ou homosexuelle hommes, mais je me demandais à quel pourcentage ou à quel degré il y a le risque de transmission [entre femmes] à ce moment-là.

(Q: Do you have any questions in particular concerning sexually transmitted infections, are there any things ... ?

R: Well, I was asking myself if there is a real risk, I don't think there's a high risk in terms of bisexuality between women, in any case less than in a heterosexual or male homosexual relation I imagine, but I was asking myself what percentage or to what degree there is a risk of transmission [between women].)

Yet this lack of knowledge of HIV and STD transmission among bisexual women is not due to their lack of effort to inform themselves. Indeed, participants recounted numerous anecdotes in which they could not receive information that was adapted specifically to women – even when they asked for such details from doctors and service providers working in the field of HIV and STDs.

Moi personnellement j'ai eu l'expérience de demander a mon médecin de famille ... Comment est-ce que je peux prévenir les MTS advenant que euh j'ai une relation sexuelle avec une femme? J'ai eu aucune réponse ... Il a pas répondu. Il m'a simplement dit courtois ..., euh, de façon courtoise la ... de, de consulter ma gynécologue. Et quand j'ai posé la question a ma gynécologue, j'ai pas eu de réponse claire comme telle. Elle m'a parlé du condom féminin … Mais c'est tout. J'ai jamais su comment ça se pose, comment ça marche, ça se trouve où, est-ce que ça coûte cher …

(Personally I've had the experience of asking my family doctor, 'How can I prevent STDs if I am with a woman?' I didn't get any answer. He didn't answer. He simply politely told me to consult my gynaecologist. And when I asked my gynaecologist, I didn't get a clear answer. She spoke to me about the female condom. But that's all. I never knew how to put it in, if it works, where to get it, does it cost a lot …)

Despite a concerted effort to obtain accurate information about how to protect herself and her partners from the transmission of STDs, this woman was unable to have her questions answered clearly after consulting two service providers, one of whom is an expert in women's health. When information was available, it was either exclusive to heterosexual relations or it addressed only men's bodies. The woman in the following quotation analyses the ways in which the information she was given about HIV and STDs did not consider women's realities:

La majorité des fois où il y avait des problèmes, c'est que la, la documentation qu'ils me donnaient c'était pour des hommes. Fait qu'il y en avait pas pour les femmes, mais ils me disaient ce que j'ai euh … ben euh tu sais euh … prends ça, lis ça, ça s'applique pas mal aux femmes aussi. Mais c'était pas, c'était pour les hommes … Mais c'était pour les hommes, tu sais. Ça s'appliquait pas à moi. C'est, c'est le seul trouble que j'ai eu … Puis euh … ici à Montréal un moment donné on a demandé euh de faire un, une soirée pour, de … pour nous en apprendre plus sur les … les contraceptifs. Pis le gars qui est arrivé de … de Séro-Zéro euh il nous a donné uniquement, uniquement des contraceptifs pour hommes, uniquement.

(Most times when there were problems, it's that the documentation that they gave me was for men. There wasn't any for women. They told me, 'Well, you know, take this, read this, it pretty much applies to women as well.' But it wasn't, it was for men. It was for men, you know. It didn't apply to me. That's the only trouble I've had. And here in Montréal at a certain time we asked to do an evening, so that we could learn more about contraceptives. And the guy who came from Séro-Zéro only gave us contraception for men, only.)

To receive a pamphlet that contains information only about men's bodies, with the advice that it's 'pretty much the same thing' for women, illustrates the manner in which many service providers do not understand the importance of attending to the specificity of women's bodies in health. Symptoms, treatment, and transmission of HIV and STDs are not the same for women and men, and as such it is insufficient to offer information concerned exclusively with men. This particular anecdote brings to light the ways in which knowledge determines the kind of information available. A knowledge framework that considers only men within HIV prevention, such as the one operating within the particular AIDS organization cited above, makes it extraordinarily difficult for women to locate the information they require.

Content Desired for Inclusion in Educational Campaigns

Having discussed some of the principal gaps in knowledge about HIV and STD transmission, participants outline what kind of content is needed to make prevention materials more relevant, particularly for bisexual women. The inclusion of women in educational campaigns directed to 'men who have sex with men' was raised as important in being able to reach men who have sex with both men and women:

> Je suis pas vraiment renseignée. Euh c'est peut-être euh ... Comme un, un homme qui est aux hommes, qui va coucher avec une femme. Il y a même pas des ... j'ai, j'ai même pas vu de renseignements sur ça là.

> (I'm not really informed. It's maybe that, like a man who is with a man, who will sleep with a woman. There aren't even any ... I've never seen any information about that.)

This woman cites an important gap in current HIV education, one that is implicitly gendered. By including women within the visual images and information of HIV and STD campaigns, she suggests a way to intervene in the current situation. A change in the content of HIV education, then, can change its audience, as well as its impact on behaviour.

In a manner parallel to the data presented in the previous chapter, participants cited a need for practical information about the transmission of HIV and STD between women. Indeed, they underlined a contradiction in the field: either women who have sexual relations with other women are completely ignored (which is generally the case), or else there is a recognition such transmission is possible, but without any kind of detailed discussion:

> But just to try and understand what the actual risks ... Or, at the very least to take existing information and compile it somewhere ... accessible, in ... such a fashion that it makes sense, and that you can explain to people what they're doing ... Because, you know, on the one hand you've got the pretty demonstrable fact that girl-on-girl sex is not generally high risk ... Right? Because otherwise, the lesbians would have been decimated by HIV too, and we're just not ... And then you've got the, sort of, the message that I've heard any time I've found anything about lesbians and STIs, and it's basically sort of around the idea that ... we don't know ..., but we know that lesbians are also affected.

This woman is clear about the kind of practical information she requires: a clear overview of the risks for STD transmission between women, as well as the concrete actions she can take to prevent such transmission.

Content of HIV and STD education that is adapted to bisexuals needs to move beyond a focus on penetration, according to our interviewees:

> R: But in mainstream literature, beyond the condom it's like, 'Oh what if you don't use a condom?' So it's kind of limiting in that sense, I think.
> Q: So you think stuff that might address other methods besides condoms?
> R: Yeah. Like sexual health outside of sexual intercourse, basically. Yeah, it's really important for people to know.

While this respondent underlines the need for sexual health information beyond the context of penetration, the following quotation recalls earlier results about the need for education specific to group sexual activities. In speaking about several women having sexual relations with a dildo, one interviewee outlines some of the specific risks :

> Il y a des femmes tu sais, il est ... Comme ils utilisent le même vibrateur sur deux femmes, tu sais là c'est trois filles, mettons tu ... Une shot là, tu sais. Il met le condom là dessus tu sais qui, pis ils échangent, changent le condom.

> (There are women, you know, like they use the same vibrator on two women, then it's three women, you know, one shot. They put the condom on it, you know, and they change the condom.)

HIV and STD education that targets bisexual men and women, then, needs to consider issues such as group sex. With specific regard to bisexual women, this means helping people understand the risk of STD transmission among women if sex toys are shared without appropriate cleaning and protection. The absence of STD campaigns that address this question suggests that the matter of group sex has yet to be fully addressed in education. But this question is also a gendered one, since this issue affects women in particular: it is women who risk contracting STDs if their partners do not use a condom for each new sexual partner. In this regard, it is in and through the neglect of women's bodies that STD education fails to provide information on the risks associated with not changing a condom when one changes a sexual partner.

The inclusion of information that is not limited to acts of penetration was repeatedly mentioned as necessary:

> ... les risques de transmission euh pour euh autres que pénétration là ... Je trouve que, ben pour les, les moyens comme autres que pénétration c'est comme si c'est un peu flou là qu'est-ce qui, qu'est-ce qu'il y a à faire en ce cas-là là.

> (... risks of transmission other than penetration ... I find that for means other than penetration it's a bit fuzzy, what to do in those cases.)

> C'est souvent eux-autres qui, ils disent, Oui, on se protège. On se protège, il y a un condom sur le pénis. Mais, il y a plein d'autres choses à risque aussi ... Tsé, c'est ça. Focusser un peu plus là-dessus ... Tsé. C'est beau dire se protéger, mais se protéger de quoi?

> (They are often the ones who say, 'Yes, we protect ourselves. We protect ourselves, there's a condom on the penis.' But there are lots of other things at risk as well. You know, that's it. Focus a little more on that. It's all well and good to say, 'Protect yourself,' but protect yourself from what?)

This insistence on including non-penetrative sexual relations reflects the realities of sexual relations between women and current gaps in prevention information.

One of the most important questions that the women we interviewed concerns the possibility of transmission of HIV and STD during oral sex between women. Like one of the participants cited above, many women had been exposed to the idea that transmission is possible between women – although they did not get this information through a prevention campaign funded in Québec. When this reality is addressed, the general tone and orientation encourages women to use latex barriers in oral sex – to cut a condom and use it as a protective barrier, or to find and use a 'dental dam' – a piece of latex that one places over the vulva for cunnilingus.

Yet the women who were familiar with this idea expressed considerable resistance to it. As the woman cited above notes,

> On the one hand you've got the pretty demonstrable fact that girl-on-girl sex is not generally high risk ... Because otherwise, the lesbians would have been decimated by HIV too, and we're just not ...

Educational campaigns directed to women, however, do not concede this point: they frequently argue that woman-to-woman transmission of HIV and other STDs is possible, and lesbians and bisexual women therefore need to protect themselves accordingly (Gorna 1996). The message to use dental dams during oral sex is intended to have women adopt safe sexual behaviours in this regard.

Yet the logic advanced by the woman cited above is not entirely false. While the data that we have on woman-to-woman transmission are certainly distorted, there are documented cases of woman-to-woman transmission of HIV, and certainly many more cases of STD transmission. The women we interviewed did not necessarily dispute this fact, but they did seek to put it in context. They were honest in their discussions with us that using dental dams was not part of their sexual practices:

> Je suis consciente des risques, sauf que ça veut pas toujours dire que j'ai le goût de prendre la protection, tsé, parce que je le sais que ça va impliquer comme moins de plaisir ou ... Je te donne un exemple de prendre une digue dentaire avec une femme pour pas avoir d'Hépatite C ou des choses comme ça, ça me tente pas toujours ... Je sais qu'il faut le faire ... Tsé, je veux dire, j'ai été éduquée comme ça, je le sais qu'il faut le faire. Sauf que ça veut pas dire que c'est toujours intéressant à le faire.
>
> (I'm aware of the risks, except that that doesn't always mean that I want to use protection, you know, because I know that will mean less pleasure. I'll give you an example of a dental dam with a woman to not get Hepatitis C

or those kinds of things, I don't always want to do it. I know you have to. You know what I mean. I was educated like that, I know what to do. But that doesn't mean that it's always interesting to do.)

More than just an individual choice, the women we interviewed noted that this was not a practice common among women who have sexual relations with women.

> R : Et j'avais vu aussi … Ah! Un flash qui me revient euh … à *Sexe et confidences* euh … Louise-Andrée Saulnier qu'elle s'appelle … Un espèce … ben pas espèce, un morceau de Saran Wrap pour faire l'amour à une femme. Je m'étais dit, 'Ben là, je pense pas que ça va être populaire ça.'
> Q : [*rires*] C'est pas très, très érotique.
> R : Non. T'as-tu déjà entendu parler de ça?
> Q : Oui.
> R : Il y a des femmes qui t'ont parlé de ça?
> Q : Oui.
> R : Non, mais tsé elle se découpait un carré là.
> Q : Oui.
> R : Tsé, comme pour emballer ton morceau de viande.
> Q : Oui.
> R : Pis elle avait comme [*inaudible*], un plastique à mettre dessus [*inaudible*], t'es tu malade toi là! Voyons donc! Et il y a aussi un autre espèce de, de … un peu comme chez le dentiste, je pense, que tu peux mettre sur la vulve, il me semble. Écoute, ça te rappelle chez le dentiste.
> Q : Non.
> R : Je connais pas personne qui fait ça.
> Q : Hm-hm.
> R : Remarque, je suis dans les fera pas là, mais.
> Q : Hm-hm.
> R : Mais moi je le ferais pas.

> (R: And I also saw … a flash that's just come to me … on *Sexe et confidences*, Louise-Andrée Saulnier she's called … a sort of piece of Saran Wrap to make love to a woman. I said to myself, 'Well I don't think that's going to be very popular.'
> Q: [*laughs*] It's not very erotic.
> R: No. Have you ever heard of that?
> Q: Yes.
> R: There are women who spoke with you about that?

Q: Yes.

R: But you know, she cut out a square.

Q: Yes.

R: To wrap up your piece of meat.

Q: Yes.

R: And she had a [*inaudible*], plastic to put on top. Are you crazy? Oh, my God! There was also this other type of thing, a little bit like at the dentist, that I think you put on top of the vulva. Anyway, it reminds you of being at the dentist.

Q: No.

R: I don't know anyone who does this.

Q: Hm-hm.

R: Listen, I'm in the 'wouldn't do it' but …

Q: Hm-hm.

R: But I wouldn't do it.)

The acknowledgment that few women use latex barriers in oral sex, and that the risks of HIV transmission during oral sex between women remain relatively low (though not non-existent), raise critical questions about how to develop meaningful prevention. While campaigns that encourage women to use latex barriers are certainly useful for getting women to think about their sexual health, the women we interviewed stated quite clearly that they would not adopt such a practice. In this regard, such educational campaigns risk alienating the very women to whom they are directed (Gorna 1996).

The complexity of these issues are discussed in detail by Robin Gorna. Writing from the British context, she recounts one HIV prevention campaign directed to women who have sex with women. Having reviewed the virological and epidemiological evidence, the health promotion planners did not see significant evidence of the risk of HIV transmission during oral sex among women. Furthermore, Gorna raises an important point about comparative education. If there is a significant risk of HIV transmission during oral sex on a woman, and if one needs to use a dental dam to prevent such transmission, then this information should be included not only in campaigns directed to women who have sex with women, but indeed within heterosexual HIV education as well. Given the review of scientific data, as well as the absence of encouragement to use of dental dams within education directed to heterosexual men, the campaign did not make recommendations for women to use latex barriers during oral sex.

Gorna documents negative reactions to the campaign from AIDS activists and educators, primarily from the United States, who advocated that prevention education on oral sex between women *must* encourage women to use latex barriers. Gorna's argument is especially interesting because she unpacks the manner in which this discourse is prevalent in the United States, as well as in countries heavily influenced by American HIV/AIDS policy and approaches to prevention.

In chapter 7 on action, we will return to this debate on transmission of HIV through oral sex between women and will discuss how we decided to address this issue. Here, we outline the fact that the women we spoke with who were aware of dental dams as a safe sex practice told us frankly that they would not adopt such a practice and that it was not in use among women who have sex with women. That said, the women we interviewed also wanted to have more clear information on the possibility of transmitting HIV and STDs between women. How to solve such an apparent contradiction will be explored in greater depth when we present the educational materials that we developed as part of this research.

Conclusion

Our data provide compelling evidence that there are gendered elements to the content of HIV and STD prevention education in Québec. Campaigns often overlook women entirely, whether as heterosexual women, as female partners of bisexual men, or as women who have sexual relations with women. Participants in our study indicate that they could not find the information they needed to prevent the transmission of HIV and STDs, especially concerning sexual relations between women, even when they made concerted efforts to seek it out. The men and women we interviewed offer more than mere documentation of the absence of women in most HIV education (although such evidence is important). They provide sophisticated analysis of the underlying causal factors at work in the exclusion of women from HIV education. In particular, our respondents examine the ways in which a bisexual person imagined in public health is always considered to be a bisexual man. Here, participants underline the ways in which public health 'knowledge' about bisexuals is implicitly gendered. Furthermore, the data cited in this chapter compel a reconsideration of the ways in which epidemiology and public health minimize the risk of transmission of HIV and STDs between women. Sometimes this occurs through neglect, as when women are not even considered in educational campaigns. In other instances, this functions through a reluctance to consider the scientific evidence in question, as when public health planners do not provide adequate attention to the issue of transmission of STDs and HIV between women. The people we interviewed challenge this kind of knowledge and remind us that they are located elsewhere and otherwise in relation to mainstream public health knowledge. Many – indeed, most – of our female participants did not have appropriate knowledge of what they could do to protect themselves against HIV and STD transmission among women. Furthermore, some people also had personal knowledge that STD and HIV transmission between women is possible. They hold such knowledge despite the lack of education on this issue. This disjuncture between the knowledge of everyday people and that of public health is, as we have shown, organized in relation to gender. The knowledge produced and advanced within public health education reflects the experience and world view of men, since the HIV and STD education that is offered does not address women's health issues comprehensively.

These reflections on the line of fault of HIV and STD knowledge and its gendered dimensions can assist us further in our analysis of how institutions function – the way they organize their work, and the people they exclude (though perhaps unwittingly). In chapter 2, we examined the specific ways in which the administrative apparatus of HIV funding is put together. We considered how the funding of HIV education programs is organized according to a logic of 'specific populations.' In that chapter, we argued that this kind of framework recognizes only certain realities and populations and that people who have sexual relations with both men and women are not well served by it. The data presented in this chapter confirm this argument, since they clearly show how and why many people with both male and female partners cannot access the HIV and STD prevention information they require. Yet the results of our research also suggest that, by organizing HIV funding according to a logic of specific populations, it is more than bisexual men and women who have been excluded. Many of our interviewees stated that they had not seen any kind of heterosexually oriented prevention materials. Moreover, they noted that HIV education in Montréal is located primarily in certain geographic locations (notably the gay village) and lamented that little or no prevention information is distributed in mainstream sites. Throughout, they underline the manner in which an absence of HIV education in the mainstream reflects gender bias, since women are not included in prevention targeted to gay men.

This data tell us something about the kinds of HIV education to which everyday people have access, as well as how women are excluded from it. Yet it also needs to be situated within a broader institutional context. Interviewees report they see little heterosexual education, and little outside the gay village. If one considers the priorities and populations named within the funding of HIV, the content (gay male) and distribution (gay village) of HIV education can be understood more clearly. Funding envelopes like the Specific Populations Fund organize themselves according to 'priority populations.' In order to obtain funding for HIV education, organizations that apply for funds need to target one of the populations considered to be 'at risk' for HIV transmission (with some limited provisions for 'cross-cutting populations'). Within this logic, there is little place for HIV education programs that target the mainstream. Rather, programs that focus on a particular category of people (e.g., prisoners, gay men, injection drug users) are given priority. To be sure, there are good reasons to organize HIV funding in this manner, especially given limited financial resources. But the data we present here caution us against thinking that such a strategy is necessarily the most effective, since we show how everyday people do not have access to the basic prevention information they require, as well as how institutional knowledge and education about HIV exclude women implicitly and explicitly. Indeed, the weaknesses of a 'specific population' approach to HIV and STD education is borne out in recent data on STD rates within the city of Baltimore.

In an epidemiological study of STDs among different populations, researchers provide an overview of STD rates within different communities, such as gay men, sex workers, and injection drug users (Wilgis 2008). When one examines the data over time, one can observe the positive impact of STD prevention programs targeted to specific populations. For example, STD prevention was conducted among both sex workers and gay men. Rates of STD infection fell during this period, illustrating the success of such prevention initiatives. Yet the data collected by the research team also contain important information about more 'mainstream' populations. While STD infection rates fell among some 'specific populations' that had been targeted for education (sex workers and gay men), infection rates rose significantly among heterosexuals in the same period. This information tells us that, by focusing exclusively on 'specific populations,' HIV and STD prevention can ignore some of the sites where rates and incidence of infection are the highest. Furthermore, such research suggests that prevention resources ought not to be allocated exclusively according to rates of infection in populations with high incidence and prevalence, since the goal of prevention is also to keep infection rates down.

The data from this study in Baltimore force a reconsideration of the logic of 'specific populations' that underpins the funding of HIV prevention initiatives in Canada. In a similar way, the voices of the men and women in our study remind us of the consequences of forgetting to address the mainstream: everyday people do not have access to the basic information they need to protect themselves and each other. In this chapter, we have documented some of these main gaps in information and have analysed how public health knowledge about HIV and STD transmission excludes women. Our research results, then, ought to be interpreted broadly – we are not making the case simply for funding bisexual-specific HIV prevention programs. After careful analysis of our interview data, we argue for the importance of integrating bisexual realities within more general HIV prevention – a position that points out the difficulties of funding mainstream HIV education within an institutional context that organizes itself according to certain recognized populations. In this regard, rather than simply adopting a 'me-too' logic for bisexuals and HIV prevention, our work suggests, more broadly, the importance of rethinking the current framework (population health) for understanding and organizing our response to this epidemic.

Our participants recount extraordinary difficulties in obtaining relevant and accurate information about HIV and STD transmission. The barriers in finding information adapted to their specific lives belies a broader challenge of being able to access good health services, since *information* about health is facilitated through *services* in particular. While obstacles in health services have certainly been raised in the present chapter, we have not yet offered sustained reflection on this relation between access to information and access to services. We turn to this question in this next chapter, in order to understand more clearly the problems faced by people who have sexual relations with both men and women. Attention to this problematic can elucidate how and why people cannot obtain the information they require, as well as what can be done about it.

6 'And That's a Big Gap, I Think': Linking HIV/STD Education and Services

In chapter 5, we cited the experiences of people who could not obtain the information they needed about HIV and STD transmission. Indeed, many of our participants made great efforts to find such knowledge. They consulted numerous service providers and asked them questions specific to their sexual lives and concerns, such as modes of transmission between women. Despite these initiatives, more often than not people still did not have answers to their questions. While such a situation certainly tells us something about the problems people have in obtaining relevant, accurate information, it also reveals broader difficulties in access to services. Challenges in accessing services are well illustrated in the anecdote (previously cited) of one woman who asked for relevant STD information from her doctor, was referred to her gynaecologist, was still unable to get the information she needed from her gynaecologist, and received no further referral to services.

Our data reveal that this situation is, alas, common – especially for women. Furthermore, our analysis of the interviews reveals an important finding: access to information is intimately linked to access to services. In this chapter, we explore this nexus of information/services in greater depth. Drawing on our interviews and relevant social scientific studies, we consider some of the main problems faced by people who have sexual relations with both men and women in finding relevant information about their sexual lives. We move from identifying this problem to analysis of its cause, which is to say, how access to quality information is dependent on good access to health institutions. Furthermore, we consider some of the suggestions put forward by participants that would improve access to health information and institutions, with a specific attention to questions of HIV and STDs.

Linking Education and Services

Our participants offered a keen analysis of some of the systemic and structural reasons why people have poor access to information. The people we interviewed cited the need to be able to evaluate information about HIV, STDs, and sexual health. Yet at the same time, they noted that in many instances, they did have access to certain kinds of information (albeit not, as we have seen, information adapted to bisexual or swinger realities). The difficulty, then, was in being able to make sense of such information and in being able to use it effectively in their everyday lives. As one interviewee puts it, access to information is not necessarily a solution:

> C'est comme ... OK, des pamphlets ça peut t'informer mais ça va pas euh ... régler, si t'as un problème ça va pas te ... t'aider à trouver comme la solution tsé. Pis j'avais déjà essayé de, d'aller faire un test du sida, mais je le savais pas où ... J'ai essayé d'aller au CLSC pis là je ... ça marchait pas comme, pis il fallait aller voir le médecin avant pis ça me tentait pas. Fait que des fois c'est un peu dur d'aller chercher le ... Ben en fait d'avoir la solution. Parce que t'as plein d'informations mais quand tu veux avoir la solution où, tsé ... vraiment, qu'on puisse t'aider, ben là c'est peut-être un peu plus difficile.

> (It's like ... OK, pamphlets that can give you information but it won't solve ... if you have a problem, it won't help you find the solution, you know. I once tried to do an AIDS test, but I didn't know where to go. I tried to go to the CLSC and then it didn't work. I had to see the doctor and I didn't want to. So sometimes it's hard to find the ... well to find the solution. Because you can have all kinds of information, but when you want to have the solution where, you know, they can help you, well that's maybe a bit more difficult.)

Such difficulties in finding a 'solution' was echoed by a number of different participants:

> Peut-être que ça rejoint pas assez les gens ça parce que ... je sais pas euh ... On dirait qu'on a l'information mais qu'on n'est pas capable d'y ... de trouver l'endroit euh spécial ... Spécifique. Tsé, mettons, t'as euh ... je sais pas comment dire. Mais on dirait qu'il y a plein d'information mais que tu peux pas y aller.

(Maybe it's doesn't reach enough people because, I don't know … It's like we have the information but we can't find the place, the specific place. You know, I don't know how to say it. It's like there is lots of information but you can't go there.)

Interviewees claimed, then, that what was needed was not simply access to information, but access to sexual health services more generally:

Q: Tu penses qu'il n'y a pas assez de ressources?
R: C'est ça. Peut-être qu'il y a assez d'informations mais que on n'a pas, on, on sait pas qu'elle est là. C'est peut-être plus ça. Tu sais, c'est le moyen de le savoir où est-ce qu'elle est.

(Q: You don't think there are enough resources?
R: That's it. Maybe there is enough information but we don't have … we don't know where it is. It's more that. You know, it's the means of knowing where it is.)

Ben il faudrait aller voir la personne ressource. Où la trouver? Bonne question [rires].

(Well, you have to go see the right resource person. Where to find them? Good question [laughs].)

C'est ça des fois, tu sais, les renseignements sont … comment je dirais ça donc? Quelqu'un qui connaît pas ça pis que … je sais pas moi, qu'il se débrouille pas icitte en ville là, qui fait rien … Il trouvera pas ce qu'il a besoin de trouver là. C'est comme quelqu'un qui tombe dans la rue, qui a jamais été dans la rue. Ben … il saura pas où est-ce qu'ils sont les organismes. Mais c'est pareil pour la personne qui, qui commence là, pis qui … Qui veut avoir des renseignements. Mais là ils savent pas où est-ce que c'est là, il faut que tu te renseignes pis là … des fois ça prend deux, trois places avant qu'ils te donnent la bonne place à aller, tu sais … C'est ça que je s …, que je voulais dire tout à l'heure par euh … par en mettre plus d'endroits spécifiques pour ça là, tu sais.

(That's it sometimes, you know, the information is, how can I say that? Someone who doesn't know this, and who, I don't know, who doesn't figure it out for herself here in the city. She won't find what she needs to find. It's like someone who ends up on the street, who was never on the street. He won't know where the organizations are. Well, it's the same for the person who starts and who ... who wants to have information. But they don't know where to go. Is it there? You have to find out, and sometimes it takes two or three places before they give you the right place to go, you know. That's what I was trying to say a moment ago. Put more places specific for that, you know.)

In all of these quotations, the interviewees underline the need to link education to services. They maintain that when one is motivated to act on sexual health, often one actually needs sexual health services – an STD check-up, an HIV test, or information on contraception. Yet sexual health educational initiatives have limited themselves to 'education' in a narrow sense, such as encouraging people to use condoms to protect themselves against HIV and STDs. While certainly preferable to no sexual health education whatsoever, such an approach does not actually facilitate people's access to sexual health services, and as such may not affect their behaviour. The participants in our study indicated that they wanted improved access to sexual health services, because this would in turn help them evaluate the contradictory information available and would increase the likelihood of adopting safe sexual behaviours. In concrete terms, they suggested educational initiatives that included a phone number and a website so that people could then access relevant sexual health services. If people need services when they are particularly concerned about HIV and or STDs, it is appropriate to ensure that prevention information and sexual health services are linked. This conjuncture of information and services suggests a new way to think about doing HIV prevention. As we discussed in chapters 4 and 5, questions of information are in turn related to knowledge itself – how knowledge frameworks determine the content of education, the individuals to be targeted, the types of sexual activities addressed, and the places of distribution. To suggest that prevention information be linked to health services compels the creation of a knowledge framework different from the one enacted to date within Canadian HIV prevention (Mykalovskiy et al. 2009).

This insistence on linking HIV education and services is both instructive and important. It brings to light how people negotiate educational campaigns and the ways in which people require good access to health services in order to properly evaluate and act on health information. Although such a position makes sound logical and intuitive sense, it is remarkable nonetheless, particularly when one considers that most HIV education is not situated within a broader context of sexual health services. Moreover, this insight is instructive because it highlights the manner in which people use, or disregard, the educational campaigns directed to them. While this research project began with the simple question of asking people about the kinds of HIV information they need, the results demonstrate that *how* that information is organized (within an education/services nexus) is as important as the *content* of the education itself. In this regard, our research offers some important data for understanding the ways in which access to health care institutions is a necessary precondition of successful educational initiatives.

Given the central role of access to sexual health services in effective HIV and STD education, the next section of this chapter examines the difficulties our participants express within health care services.

Access to Health Care Services for Bisexual Men and Women

Within Québec, empirical research demonstrates some of the particular health challenges faced by individuals who have sexual relations with both men and women. Within a large-scale survey of health care and social service needs in Québec, the Institut de Statistique du Québec discovered that bisexual men and women confront numerous difficulties in their overall social and health needs. Compared to other sexual minorities (lesbians and gay men), bisexuals indicated less social integration and stronger feelings of isolation (ISQ 1998). Such social alienation manifests itself at the individual level as well, with bisexuals experiencing a rate of attempted suicide significantly higher than either heterosexuals or lesbians and gay men (ISQ). Bisexual women have higher rates of alcoholism than either lesbians or heterosexual women, and bisexuals overall report lower revenues than other sexual minorities in Québec (ISQ). Moreover, Canadian data reveal that bisexual men and women are more frequently victims of violence than either lesbians and gay men or heterosexuals (Statistics Canada 2008). These data, then, tell us about the ways in which bisexual men and women are marginalized in Canadian and Québec society, as well as how such marginalization has negative consequences for their health. While the studies cited above provide an overview of the situation, empirical research conducted in Ontario indicates the poor access of bisexual men and women to health care and social services (Dobinson et al. 2005). Negative attitudes towards bisexuals, misconceptions about bisexuality, and service providers ill-equipped to serve bisexual clients represent some of the biggest challenges in this domain. Bisexual men and women in Canada have difficulty finding health services that are non-judgmental, relevant, and comprehensive (Dobinson et al.). Our study builds on these research findings and provides a specific analysis of the problems bisexual men and women in Montréal face in accessing sexual health services.

In certain instances, difficulties in accessing services were not specific to bisexuality per se, but rather reflect people's lack of knowledge of available resources. One man interviewed, for example, recounts the challenges he encountered in finding services to deal with genital warts:

> Voilà une couple d'années la euh ... il y avait, même il faut dire que je me suis retrouvé chez un gynécologue la ... Parce que j'avais une infection euh ... c ..., c'était des condylomes la que j'avais attrapés ... il [mon médecin] savait rien dans ça ... C'est une amie de fille qui m'avait euh présenté a son gynécologue ... Mais je me suis informé euh ... c'est elle qui m'a informé de ça la.

> (A couple of years ago, I have to tell you that I found myself at the gynaecologist. Because I had an infection, I had gotten genital warts. My doctor didn't know anything about it. It's a female friend of mine that referred me to her gynaecologist. But I informed myself, it's her that informed me about that.)

Unaware of existing services in the field of sexual health, this man appealed to his personal network of friends to be able to access relevant health care. This experience illustrates the tremendous amount of work people must do to obtain services and further confirms the ways in which current sexual health education is disconnected from services.

In addition to general difficulties locating relevant services (such as in the anecdote recounted above), participants in our study reported that service providers had negative attitudes about bisexuality. In particular, many providers held the idea that the 'promiscuous' nature of bisexuality puts bisexual men and women at increased risk for infection with HIV or other STDs. One woman, who was open with her service provider about having multiple stable partners simultaneously, was informed that she could reduce her risk of STDs if she reduced her number of partners. The woman identifies herself as polyamorous, meaning that she has the potential of being involved with more than one partner at the same time. Polyamory underlines the committed nature of such relationships and is to be distinguished from more casual encounters with multiple partners: one may have several partners, but these are the same people on a regular basis.

> I'm also polyamorous and I had an awful experience with trying to get this through to doctors that ... She said that oh, she basically told me, 'You should try to limit your partners.' That's not something you tell someone who's a polyamorist, and I tried to explain to her that having three consistent partners for six months is not necessarily any more dangerous than having three within a six-month time span.

Here, the service provider's lack of understanding of polyamory meant that the specific articulation of 'multiple partners' was understood to be similar to having multiple casual sexual partners. Moreover, the doctor's advice was clearly not adapted to this woman's sexual lifestyle, since she was already open about having numerous partners. The anecdote is instructive, however, because it illustrates the ways in which misconceptions of sexuality can inform the kinds of services delivered.

While in some instances misconceptions about bisexuality were clearly visible, in other cases discrimination is more implicit:

> There's definitely a judgment of whether it's someone I know, or someone I'm dating. I can just see the judgment in the doctor's face when I say, like, 'Oh yeah, we've been together a couple of times, but it's nothing serious,' and she's automatically like, 'Oh, I know that you don't have a job, I know that you have sex with random people that you're not really dating; you must have really low self-esteem.' And I'm just like, 'No, low self-esteem is not the problem.'

Stereotypes of bisexuals as non-committal, unreliable, and sexually insatiable were cited as common attitudinal barriers within health care services among service providers. Moreover, many participants underscored the fact that their particular health needs – notably mental health needs – were inextricably linked to questions of sexuality, although they could not necessarily be reduced to them:

> Je buvais beaucoup aussi. J'avais commencé à boire parce que j'étais comme vraiment stressée euh. Je me disais, Ah, je suis tannée d'être

toujours euh ... tsé comme marginale. Tsé, j'ai toujours été marginale, point. Mais là c'était encore plus.

(I was drinking a lot. I started to drink because I was really stressed. I said to myself, Oh, I'm tired of always being, you know, marginal. You know, I was always marginal, period. But then it was even more.)

Mais tsé moi c'est pas mes expériences bisexuelles qui m'ont ... Qui m'ont menée dans les urgences ou quoi que ce soit ... Sauf que je sais que c'est, c'est relié. Moi j'ai, j'étais avec des personnes dans ce temps-là [de consommation de drogues], qui, qui étaient, qui étaient bisexuelles aussi pis les gens ... En général euh ne se protégaient pas vraiment. Euh pis avec la drogue aussi tsé tu ... Peut-être, je le sais pas comment ça se passe euh ... Moi ça a toujours été dans un, un contexte de drogue mes expériences bisexuelles ou presque.

(But you know, for me, it wasn't my bisexual experiences that led me to the emergency room or anything. Except that I know that they're linked. I was with people then [during a period of drug use] who were bisexual, and people didn't really protect themselves. And you know with the drugs too. Maybe, I don't know how it works ... my bisexual experiences were always within a drug context or almost always.)

These quotations offer qualitative data that confirm the finding of the Québec Health Survey which indicates the isolation, and alcohol and drug use among bisexual men and women in Québec. Service provision to members of this population, then, needs to consider the complex ways in which sexuality, drug use, and social integration intersect. In all cases, participants claimed the need for specific training on bisexuality, as well as training that would situate bisexuality within a broader context of health care needs:

I don't know if you're planning on doing some kind of outreach with doctors or with health care professionals, or the very basics ... There's so many things they need to get trained about.

The need to train doctors and health care service providers on the specific realities of bisexual men and women emerges as an important recommendation of this research, itself linked to a broader analysis of the ways in which bisexuals are marginalized within health care institutions. While the need to provide further education on bisexualities is generalized across our research interviews, our research has also uncovered questions of access to health care and social services specific to swingers. The next section of this chapter explores this question in greater depth.

Swingers: Access to Condoms

As outlined in chapter 3 with regards to methodology, this research project sought to interview a wide diversity of people who have sexual relations with both men and women in Montréal. As part of such an objective, the project included targeted recruitment within swinger establishments. The term *swinger* refers to heterosexual couples who exchange sexual partners occasionally or regularly.

Within Québec, swingers have great visibility. In the late 1990s, police raided certain swinger clubs, parties, and events where couples met and exchanged sexual partners. Owners and patrons were charged under the laws related to prostitution in Canada, notably the bawdy house laws (operating a bawdy house for the owners, and being a found-in within a common bawdy house for the patrons). These raids had extensive media coverage in the Québec press, from talk shows to daily newspapers like *Le Journal de Montréal* (Hamel 2003). Importantly, however, owners and managers of swinger establishments challenged such persecution. They took the government to court and proceeded all the way to the Supreme Court of Canada. In a landmark decision in 2005, the Supreme Court of Canada acknowledged the legality of swinger establishments in the country (R. v. Labaye 2005). Throughout this process, swinger culture has remained within the public eye.

The Supreme Court decision has had a positive impact on the visibility and development of swinger culture in Montréal. The clear legal situation has meant that more people are comfortable frequenting such businesses, since they do not fear police repression.[1] The greater Montréal region has a wide market of swinger establishments: mixed saunas, clubs, a boat cruise, and private evenings. The number and diversity of activities attest to the vibrancy of this sexual culture in and around the city.

With regards to health services, and HIV prevention initiatives in particular, our research demonstrates that in certain instances, swingers do not have easy access to condoms – primary prevention materials in protection against HIV. The people interviewed describe the lack of condoms in certain establishments:

Écoutez, on rentre dans le club euh il y a même pas de, de ... pas de machine a condom, il a pas de plaquette d'information sur le VIH, le, la chlamydia, la gonorrhée, etc. Donc on dit rien, il y a, en fait j'ai été euh ... quelques fois dans des saunas gais et c'est les seuls endroits ou on vous donnait une serviette, un condom pis une clé pour votre placard. Dans un sauna ..., dans un sauna mixte ou un club mixte, rien, rien du tout.

(Listen, you go in the club there aren't even any ... not even any condom distribution machines, no posters on HIV, chlamydia, gonorrhoea, etc. So nothing is said. There is, in fact I was in, sometimes in gay saunas and they are the only places where they give you a towel, a condom, and a key for your locker. In a mixed sauna or a mixed club, nothing at all.)

Pis je crois qu'il y juste un endroit qui est [nom du club] ... qu'il y avait des condoms euh gratuits ... Les autres endroits il fallait payer des machines distributrices ou il fallait les apporter, il y en avait pas sur place directement ... Pis ça c'est un gros manque, je pense.

(And I think there's just one place which is ... where they have free condoms. The other places you have to pay distribution machines or you have to bring them. They don't have any onsite. And that's a big gap, I think.)

Interviewees noted that certain establishments did have condoms available, but that the access was limited, given their location, as well as cost:

Au sauna, euh c'est ... c'est des machines distributrices en haut dans le fond cachées. Pis euh ... une petite boîte de trois condoms c'est hyper cher, c'est extrêmement cher ... Fait que si tu les amène pas avec toi, euh il faut que t'ailles chercher l'argent dans ton casier en bas parce que t'es en serviette ... Que tu remontes, que t'ailles chercher ta boîte de condoms. Tu peux même pas la serrer nulle part parce que t'es en serviette ... pis c'est ça aussi, les places en serviette c'est que ... C'est comme l'autre fois je me, je suis allée, je me suis ramassée dans une chambre pis, « Ah merde, les condoms. On les a oublié en bas ». Là il faut retourner à la case en bas, aller chercher les condoms, remonter. Ça c'est un peu euh ... un peu plate. Tandis que dans d'autres clubs où j'ai été euh dans les, les sections où il se passait de la sexualité, il y avait des condoms partout ... Euh disponibles euh pis les gens les prenaient pis c'était ... on pige dedans pis ... facile là ... Pis quand ils sont à la vue aussi euh ça incite beaucoup les gens. Moi je dirais c'est plus ça. Ils sont là, pourquoi pas le prendre … Oui. Plus c'est facile, plus les gens euh le font.

(At the sauna … the distribution machines are up top, hidden in the back. And a little box of three condoms is super expensive, it's really expensive. So if you don't bring some with you, you have to go get your money in your locker because below you're in your towel. When you go back up, you go get your condoms. You can't even keep them anywhere because you're in a towel, and that's it too, the towel places. It's like the other time I went, I found myself in a room and, 'Oh shit, the condoms, we forgot them downstairs.' So you have to return to the locker below, go get your condoms, go back up. So it's a bit … a bit annoying. Whereas in other clubs where I've been in the sections were sex occurs, condoms are everywhere. Available, and people took them, you just grab them, it's easy. And when you can see them, that encourages people. I would say it's that. They're there, why not take them. Yes, the easier it is, the more people will do it.)

In order to improve access to condoms, the people we interviewed emphasized that condoms should be free and readily available:

Ce serait vraiment bien qu'il ait euh beaucoup plus d'endroits ou les condoms seraient gratuits … Tu sais parce qu'ils y a énormément des gens qui ont des relations sexuelles non protégées parce que ils en ont pas, ils ont, ils ont pas de condom sur eux.

(It would be really great if there were lots more places where the condoms were free. You know, because there are lots of people who have unprotected sexual relations because they don't have a condom on them.)

Juste le fait que ça soit gratis, crime ça va aider le monde a … a faire attention.

(Just the fact that it's free, God, that will help people pay attention.)

D'obliger les clubs ou euh que, que le gouvernement donne des condoms euh gratuitement en quantité.

(Require that the clubs or that the government give free condoms in large quantities.)

These problems in access to condoms were confirmed within our participant observation in swinger establishments, as well as our conversations with business managers and owners. In the initial phases of our research, we contacted different managers and owners to explain our research and to request their assistance in recruitment of interviewees. One individual in particular expressed enthusiasm for the project and asked if we could assist in securing free and or inexpensive access to condoms. (Happily, we were able to do so, in collaboration with a local community health organization.) This request is instructive, however. It indicates that the managers and owners of some of the main swinger businesses in Montréal have virtually no relation to community-based HIV/AIDS organizations, or to the local department of public health. Despite the visibility of swingers in Québec society, and despite common knowledge that swinger businesses are by definition sites where people are sexually active, people working in HIV/AIDS prevention and public health have not thought it especially relevant to work with swinger communities in the fight against HIV and STDs and the promotion of sexual health. Our research, then, illustrates some of the surprising gaps within HIV education in Québec: one of the most visible and sexually active communities of the largest city in the province has been entirely neglected. More than twenty-five years into an epidemic, public health has not ensured that thousands of sexually active adults in Montréal have free, easy access to primary HIV and STD prevention materials and information.

The data cited above are specific to swingers and demonstrate the ways in which HIV and prevention services have yet to include populations (such as swingers) who remain unrecognized. Such barriers to health services were equally evident for the women we interviewed – a situation we consider in greater depth in the next section of this chapter.

'Et les filles?' The Lack of Sexual Health Information for Bisexual Women

In chapter 5, we examined the ways in which HIV and STD education is gendered: how a viewer of educational campaigns is assumed to be male, and how the information presented neglects to consider the range and complexities of disease transmission with regard to women's bodies, notably in sexual relations between women. Such a gender bias is, according to our interviewees, equally present within sexual health services. One woman, for example recounted the manner in which her needs were dismissed as irrelevant:

> One of them [a doctor in a clinic] mentioned that she didn't want to check me [for STDs] … She kind of was [*laughing*], she's like, 'You're a woman, you don't need this checked, or this checked, or this checked.' … I just got really angry and left [*laughing*].

Here, the idea that women who are sexually involved with other women are not at risk for HIV and STDs is taken to its logical conclusion: since, the argument goes, these women are not at risk, there is no need to test them for such conditions – even when they request it! This experience relies on the argumentation examined in previous chapters, in which epidemiology underestimates the importance of woman-to-woman transmission of STDs and HIV. Medical service providers such as the doctor cited above then appeal to such 'evidence' in order to make decisions about the kinds of service they offer. Here, we witness the manner in which frameworks of knowledge inform what kinds of services are available.

Difficulties women experience accessing information are not limited to individual cases. Indeed, interviewees offered analysis of the manner in which the organizations working in the field of HIV/AIDS themselves both reflect and constitute specific gender bias. The ways that organizations did not address women's needs was well summarized by one woman:

> Puis euh … ici à Montréal un moment donné on a demandé euh de faire un, une soirée pour, de … pour nous en apprendre plus sur les … les contraceptifs. Pis le gars qui est arrivé de … de Séro-Zéro euh il nous a donné uniquement, uniquement des contraceptifs pour hommes, uniquement.

> (And here in Montréal at a certain moment, we asked to have an evening to learn more about contraception. And the guy came from Séro-Zéro, he only gave us contraceptives for men, only.)

The woman here is referring specifically to an introductory workshop on HIV and STDs that was organized by the community group Bi Unité Montréal (BUM) in 2005. Her analysis of the situation was confirmed in our field research, as some of us attended the workshop as participants and organizers.[2] Indeed, the contraceptive materials distributed were condoms – and male condoms at that. The workshop facilitator had participants touch and manipulate different kinds of condoms for men, yet at no point did he distribute a female condom. Such an absence reflects a general lack of attention to women's issues. Yet it is particularly glaring, given that female condoms are especially relevant as a method of HIV and STD prevention for women who are allergic to latex (they are made from polyurethane). Specific information about sexual practices also considered only men's bodies: the facilitator spoke of special lubricant that was available for fisting but was referring in particular to anal fisting of men. He did not discuss vaginal fisting and what lubricants could be used if necessary, as well as their potential impact on vaginal health and the possibility of a yeast infection. Similarly, participants were told that one of the symptoms of syphilis was a chancre on the penis, but they were not given the information that such a chancre can also manifest itself on the lips of the vagina, as well as in the vagina's interior. Indeed, the virtual absence of women's bodies was remarkable: not once in an educational workshop on HIV and STD transmission did the facilitator speak about menstrual blood in relation to disease transmission. Documentation distributed at the workshop further assumed a male audience, including a pamphlet with the text 'Amusez-vous gaiement' (Play gay). To distribute such information at an HIV/STD workshop for bisexual men and women indicates, in our view, a lack of reflection on the fact that the men present may have female partners, or that the women present may not even have male partners. Participants were somewhat critical of the content and approach offered in this workshop. Indeed, one woman asked the facilitator if he and his organization did HIV prevention only with men, and the answer was in the affirmative. The lack of appropriate services for women was further confirmed after the workshop, when – as these things often occur – a number of women stayed to lament the fact that they still did not have accurate information about transmission of STDs between women. Although we were there as observers and participants, in the following week we sent this kind of information on to BUM so that the group could, in turn, distribute it to its members. In this manner, our field research identified a concrete instance in which HIV and STD services offered little or nothing to women. By providing relevant information addressing women's bodies, we endeavoured to give women the information that they actively sought out and was so difficult to obtain.

Interviewees underlined that situations such as this workshop were, unfortunately, common. Our field research reveals that, in fact, members of BUM, the community organization that had invited Séro-Zéro to give this educational workshop, had asked them to come prepared to speak about HIV and STD transmission issues specific to women.[3] In a related manner, one of our participants maintains that community agencies like Séro-Zéro hold tremendous visibility in Montréal and are frequently assumed to be experts in the milieu. Yet the content and orientation of their work excludes women entirely:

Parce que dans le milieu communautaire Séro-Zéro est extrêmement présent ... A tous les événements ils sont la. Ils distribuent des préservatifs partout, partout, partout. Enfin la ou moi j'ai été disons ... Ils ont toujours, toujours, toujours été la. On leur a toujours reprogé ... , reproché pardon, la même chose, c'est que c'est très bien de distribuer des préservatifs, bravo c'est génial mais et les filles?

(Because within the community sector, Séro-Zéro is extremely present. They are at all the events. They give out condoms everywhere, everywhere. Or at least where I was, let's say ... They were always, always there. We always criticized them, for the same thing, it's really great to give out condoms, bravo, it's super, but what about the ladies?)

These specific comments about Séro-Zéro speak to much broader gaps in sexual health services. When asked where they would send someone who has sexual relations with both men and women and who needed information on HIV and STDs, our respondents noted the utter lack of available resources for women in particular:

Parce que souvent ... Aussi posée la question, « Mais qu'est-ce qu'on peut faire pour les femmes » ? ... qui viennent poser des questions, etc., etc. Ben a qui on va les référer, a quelle association? C'était ça aussi une question ...

(Because often, asked the question, 'What can we do for women?' who come to ask questions, etc. Well, to whom can we refer them, to which agency? That too is a question.)

Because, for example, if the person asking me that were a gay guy, I would probably send them to Séro-Zéro or somewhere. Because that's sort of a major organization that I know caters to exactly that group ... For girls there's just so little. Like, I did research to find it [information on STD transmission between women] and I couldn't. So I don't know where I'd send them ... I mean, in terms of sending a ... like a bi girl somewhere, to get information ... Fucked if I know.)

Indeed, the dilemma posed by the above interviewees is more than hypothetical. Having conducted research on this question since 2004, we would not have a clear organization to which we could refer bisexual women in Montréal for the sexual heath information they need to protect themselves and their partners. (We would, however, refer them to our website, www.polyvalence.ca. We discuss our website in greater depth in the next chapter.)

To consider access to health services for bisexuals, then, must necessarily mean to give attention to gender. Our research shows that women in particular are unable to access the sexual health information they require, in part because service providers underestimate their vulnerability to HIV and STDs and disregard their bodies. The invisibility of women within the knowledge we commonly have of HIV (including within scientific knowledge) in turn affects the kinds of services that are made available in the field.

Suggestions for Linking Education and Services

Having identified the ways in which poor access to health services impedes access to HIV and STD information, the men and women with whom we spoke offered concrete suggestions to link HIV/STD education and services. They wanted to be able to speak with someone in order to evaluate the information available:

On peut aller chercher un pamphlet mais c'est pas euh ... comme avoir une conversation avec quelqu'un la ... C'est pas en profondeur.

(We can get a pamphlet, but it's not like having a conversation with someone. It's not in depth.)

R : Et peut-être euh ... J'aimerais voir comme une ressource ... Soit un numéro de téléphone euh d'information.
Q : Qu'on te ... on te dirige vers quelque part où tu ...
R : Parce que ça, ça fa, ça te fait dire dans la tête : « Oh moi est-ce que je n'étais pas testée, j'ai ... que j'étais avec deux, trois différents partenaires » et puis ça te fait peur. Alors quand tu penses, quand tu en penses, tu veux demander des questions, trouver quelque part pour être testée.

(R: And maybe I'd like to have a resource. Either a telephone number ...

Q: They direct you somewhere ...

R: Because, you say to yourself, Oh, I haven't been tested, I was with two or three different partners, and then you get scared. So you think ... you think you want to ask questions, find somewhere you can get tested.)

For education to be successful, it needs to be able to help people connect to relevant services so that they can make sense of different information on HIV and STDs. Posters should include a telephone number people can call and speak with someone directly. We ought to underline here, as well, that older respondents in particular articulated a desire to be able to speak with someone directly. In this light, if one seeks to do effective HIV and STD prevention with older people, one must have a telephone information line in place. Many of our interviewees over forty stated a preference for speaking on the phone or in person with someone, as opposed to locating information on a website. Moreover, posters need to include a website that would both contain additional information and direct people to appropriate services. Without such concrete elements, our participants claimed, posters and educational materials would remain at an abstract level and would not be effective (as the data presented in chapter 4 demonstrate). To include a telephone number and website, however, would not only provide information. More importantly, such an approach would improve people's access to primary health care services. Given the difficulties bisexual men and women experience in obtaining such services, the contribution of such an approach is not to be underestimated.

In addition to these tactics of including a phone number and website on educational materials, our respondents identified clear strategies for specific services. In the case of swingers, a 'mobile unit team' that works to do prevention in swinger saunas, clubs, cruises, and private parties was cited as needed:

Je viens de penser à quelque chose ... Organiser des, des promotions pour les gens qui font des, euh, des fêtes ou des partys ou ces choses là. C'est que si vous faites un party, appelez-vous on nous envoie des condoms pis des dépliants ... Dans les milieux tu sais où est-ce qu'il se passe beaucoup de choses. Pis ce serait [rires] ce serait extrêmement bon, tu sais. Si, tu sais, vraiment si tu fais un party chez-vous t'appelles et voilà : « Moi je fais un party pis on va être euh environ tant de personnes » ... Tu sais, on t'envoie comme un ... je sais pas tu sais, un stock de ... de condoms, avec tu sais des dépliants pis des choses attrayantes, des petits, tu sais des petites bébelles, des ... pas des bébelles là mais tu sais euh ... le monde dans les partys ça se fait du fun avec des, des parapluies qu'il y a dans les drinks, fait que tu sais euh ça, ça prend pas grand chose là pour amuser les gens. Pis tu sais, ils vont s'en souvenir du condom. Donc tu sais, ça c'est ... ça, ça fonctionnerait vraiment beaucoup ... Comme un espèce de équipe mobile, c'est ça [rires].

(I just thought of something. Organize promotions for people who organize parties or evenings or those kinds of things. So if you're having a party, call and we'll give you condoms and pamphlets. You know, in the scenes where a lot is going on. That would be really good [laughs] you know. If, you know, you are having a party, you call and that's it: 'I'm organizing a party and we'll be so many people.' You know, they send you like, I don't know, a stock of condoms, with you know, pamphlets, some attractive things, little party favours, not party favours but you know ... people in parties they have fun with that, umbrellas in the drinks, so you know, it doesn't take a lot to amuse people. And you know, they're going to remember the condom. So you know, it's ... that would work really well ... Like a kind of mobile team, that's it [laughs])

This kind of 'mobile team' to do the work of HIV and STD prevention is, of course, a model that has been employed for many years in certain settings. Gay male AIDS organizations, for instance, often have a team of staff and volunteers that does outreach to bars and saunas, making sure that condoms are readily available to patrons. The suggestion put forward above is to have something similar, but adapted specifically for swingers. Moreover, given that many people may be involved in swinging activities without going to public swinger establishments (clubs and saunas), the mobile team could reach a population of sexually active people who would not be reached if prevention efforts were concentrated exclusively within commercial sites. This comment, then, reveals deep knowledge about how people organize their sexual lives and what specific type of intervention is required to reach them.

In a parallel manner, interviewees remark on the need for a vaccination campaign against hepatitis A and B:

R : Mais moi je dis, un moyen efficace, ce serait ça. Ce serait le vaccin contre l'hépatite A, B, C, ou je sais pas qu'est-ce qui ... Pourrait avoir comme vaccin là. Pis la prévention en même temps pour le VIH pis toutes ces

affaires-là pis expliquer comment est-ce que ça peut se poigner pis
tout … Tu sais, ça coûte quoi là donner un vaccin pis parler cinq minutes,
dix minutes, quinze minutes avec les personnes … T'en fais pas vingt à la
fois … T'es sûr que la personne comprend comme il faut, tu sais … C'est
ben mieux que d'arriver après pis lui dire, « Ah ben … » tu sais là … Une
petite annonce de trente secondes comme je te disais tantôt là.

Q : Oui, c'est pas assez.

R : Ça c'est pas écoeurant … Pis si la personne elle veut poser une question,
elle va poser la question à la tv? Elle peut pas là.

(R: But I say, an effective way, that's it. It would be the vaccine against hepatitis A, B, C, or I don't know what you can have as a vaccine. And HIV
prevention at the same time for all those things, and explain how they
can be caught. You know, what does it cost to give a vaccine and talk
five minutes, ten minutes, fifteen minutes with people … You don't do
twenty at the same time. You're sure that the person understands as they
should, you know. It's much better than getting there after and saying to
them, 'Oh well … ' A little thirty-second ad, as I was saying before.

Q: Yes, that's not enough.

R: That's not the bomb. And if the person wants to ask a question, is she
going to ask a question of the television? She just can't.

This interviewee envisions good access to health services as necessary
conditions for effective prevention. In contrast to generalized education
on television, a vaccination campaign against hepatitis within swinger
communities would provide an occasion for nursing personnel and
community health workers to answer questions about the transmission, symptoms, treatment, and prevention of many different STDs.
Moreover, such a strategy would fit well within the work of a 'mobile
team' cited above. A mobile team that included vaccination in its work
would provide an engaging model for access to health care more
broadly. Participants active in swinger communities further suggested
that HIV and STD transmission information could be incorporated into
regular 'Introduction to Swinging' evenings offered in Montréal. These
evenings provide an overview of the milieu for couples new to the
experience and answer any questions people may have. By integrating
content on HIV and STDs, one could ensure that many new swingers
receive the information they need from their entry into the scene.

Aside from specific services to ensure that relevant information is
distributed, participants gave critical feedback about the way in which

HIV and STD education should be organized. Here, we draw attention not so much to the content of the materials (which we examined in chapters 4 and 5) as to how education should be conceptualized, framed, and delivered. The men and women we interviewed underlined the importance of education in mainstream sites:

Dans des centres commerciaux. C'est une des meilleures places qu'ils devraient pour faire la prévention. Il devrait avoir des petites tables avec des condoms aux centres commerciaux. Parce que les jeunes le jeudi soir, c'est où ils vont? Aux centres commerciaux. Pis à neuf heures quand ils finissent, ils font quoi? Ils vont prendre une liqueur sur le coin de la patate, sur le coin, pis qu'est-ce qu'ils font après? Ben ils font leurs petites expériences sexuelles. Fait que c'est comme ça. C'est à la patate du coin qu'il faut que tu mettes de la prévention.

(In shopping centres. That's one of the best places where there should be prevention. They should have tables with condoms in the shopping centres. Because the youth on Thursday nights, where do they go? To the mall. And at 9 pm when they're done, what do they do? They're going to have a soft drink at the corner restaurant, and what are they going to do after? Well their little sexual experiences. So it's like that. It's at the corner restaurant that you have to put prevention.)

As we have seen in previous chapters, the development of education for specific populations recognized in state institutions and community organizations has meant that HIV and STD education that targets mainstream society has received less visibility than that focused on populations such as gay men. Our participants argue that they need education oriented to the mainstream, but that nonetheless acknowledges the possibility of bisexual relations and gives people the information and services they require.

To develop education that is 'mainstream' but recognizes bisexuality is easier said than done. Interviewees underline the importance of a discreet framework in which education takes place:

Arrêter de voir juste deux personnes … En voir trois ou quatre. J'aimerais ça voir euh des gens dits « normaux » … Euh je le sais pas, peut-être une … un couple de monsieur-madame tout le monde euh … j'aimerais voir la bisexualité mâle, mais tu sais pas, rien de, de, de choquant là. Tu sais euh comme euh un couple de monsieur-madame toutlemonde que le monsieur par en arrière il tient la main d'un autre homme, tu sais. Quelque chose de discret, tu sais … Mais ils se tendent pas vraiment la main un vers l'autre là … Ils se touchent pas, tu sais.

(Stop seeing just two people. See three or four. I'd like to see so-called normal people. I don't know, maybe a couple, Mr and Mrs Jones, I'd like to see male bisexuality, but you know, nothing shocking. You know, like Mr and Mrs Jones with the man behind he's holding his arm out towards the other man, you know. Something discreet, you know. But they aren't really reaching their hands towards each other. They do not touch, you know.)

Tu restes dans un quartier straight pis qu'il y a des … personnes euh homo-sexuelles, des personnes euh … bisexuelles qui viennent près de chez-toi, ben je suis certain que ces personnes là vont être tellement discrets … Que non, ça paraîtra pas … Fait que fais donc la même chose dans la publicité.

(You live in a straight neighbourhood and there are homosexual people, bisexuals that come near you. I am certain that those people are going to be so discreet so that it wouldn't be obvious. So do the same thing with the publicity.)

Mais il faudrait que, vraiment qu'il y ait deux couples dessus. Un couple à gauche, un couple à droite … Pour vraiment euh dire … même pas de mentionner échangistes, juste de voir les deux couples. Euh on saurait tout de suite que c'est deux couples qui sont échangistes, tout simple-ment … Je trouve que ce serait ou un couple avec une femme ou avec un homme … Là ce serait vraiment euh … t'aurais même pas, la, juste la photo parlerait. Sauf que quand même il faudrait que tu spécifierais plus euh … du côté euh … les MTS ou ben sur le côté VIH. Mais pas vraiment beaucoup. Juste des petites notes de rien. Mais juste la photo parlerait.

(But you'd need, really two couples on it. One couple on the left, one on the right. To really say … not even to mention swingers, just to see two couples. We would simply know right away that it's two couples who are swingers. I think that it would be either a couple with a woman or with a man. That would be really … you wouldn't even have … just the photo would speak. But you'd have to specify all the same more about STDs or HIV. But not really a lot. Just little notes. Just the photo would speak.)

In different ways, these quotations suggest possibilities for specific visual content, as well as general considerations in the orientation of prevention. A framework that remains discreet is important. This emphasis on a subtle approach is not to say, however, that such education cannot also represent relations that are same-sex, between couples, and or within a group. As the above comments make clear, the issue is how the content is packaged.

The discreet orientation of prevention materials and services within the mainstream is further important, given the stigma surrounding HIV and AIDS. Indeed, stigma remains an important obstacle to our actions and understandings of HIV/AIDS in Canada, with misconceptions about the disease, its transmission, and its treatment still common (CPHA 2005). Moreover, stigma can also prevent people from seeking out the information or services they require. The people we interviewed acknowledged these difficulties and cited examples of productive ways to organize services that help minimize stigma:

> I was just thinking, there was a counsellor at high school, and she was saying – this is just kind of random – but she was saying that she had a bunch of pamphlets and brochures and stuff and, like outside her office or right inside her office, and also, she was there, so the way she got the kids to come to her is that any time that you went there you got a candy, so you didn't go in for a brochure, so you didn't go in to talk to the counsellor, you went in to get a candy. 'Oh and by … and how was your day?' 'Well actually …' and just that approach, I just like. I was so amazed by her, for thinking of, like a way to like make it, like, 'Oh look, he's walking into the … the counsellor's office, I wonder what's wrong with him, or I wonder …' He went in for a break and a candy, you know, and I don't … just that kind of idea, like that really, that, I guess that, sums up what I think is effective, just that idea.

Related to this question of framing education discreetly, participants claim the need to avoid an identity-based approach to this education. Effective education will include information related to bisexualities, but it will not necessarily announce itself as such – for example, proclaiming that it is HIV education for bisexual men and women. One quotation explains the importance of working outside an identity-based frame:

> I think people who aren't out about it or don't identify with the dominant words used, I think often separate themselves. So they'll be like, 'Oh, I'm

not like that, I'm not gay, I just have sex with men sometimes.' So I think that can be hard. Again, I think it would be good to just talk about acts, specifically about sex and not about the kind of sex. I think even the word *bisexual* ... a lot of people don't identify with the word *bisexual*.

Indeed, many of our interviewees refused the label *bisexual* as a way to describe themselves, although they had sexual relations with both men and women. The woman cited below embodies such complex relations to the category. While she clearly acknowledges sexual relations with both men and women, she is not interested in political identity or affiliation:

Pis je suis pas axée sur euh, je suis pas une euh ... comment je dirais ça donc eh? Je suis bisexuelle ... Bon, il faut que j'embarque dans un groupe avec une étampe dans le front ... Même si j'ai pas l'étampe dans le front. C'est pas ... c'est pas ça que je veux. Je veux pas avoir une, euh, continuité. Moi, j'ai le goût d'une bonne baise, j'ai ... 'That's it.' Le lendemain, c'est autre chose ... Tsé, pis ça peut se reproduire juste dans deux mois. Pis c'est correct ... Mais j'irais pas comme ... bon ben 'je veux me tenir avec des bisexuelles' ... Non, non. Ça me tente pas là, c'est pas ça.

(And I'm not really that oriented, I'm not really that ... how can I say this? I am bisexual. So I have to join a group with a stamp on my forehead. Even if I don't have my forehead stamped. It's not ... it's not what I want. I don't want to have any follow-through. Me, I just want a good fuck, that's it. The next day, it's something else. You know, it can happen again only in two months. And it's fine. But I wouldn't go and be like, 'Well I'm going to hang out with bisexual women.' No, no. I'm not interested, it's not that.)

This quotation is important from the perspective of access to information and services. The speaker tells us, very implicitly, that she is not interested in searching out services or a community organization that specifically names itself 'bisexual.' The development of HIV education for people who have sexual relations with men and women needs to acknowledge such a complex situation. One concrete way to do this is to ensure that the information is distributed in the mainstream, outside of gay and lesbian communities:

Je connais beaucoup de bisexuelles comme moi qui se sentent pas acceptées dans le village, donc peut-être que c'est pas cibler dans le village. Peut-être euh ... ce serait plutôt dans un ... un journal euh à ... Comme le *Voir* ou le ... le *Miroir*. Peut-être un journal gratuit qui est à la portée de tous. Je pense que ça serait plus efficace.

(I know lots of bisexual women like me who do not feel accepted in the [gay] village, so maybe do not target the village. Maybe, it would be more in a newspaper like the *Voir* or the *Mirror*. Maybe a free newspaper that anyone can get. I think that would be more effective.)

I don't like to go to straight clubs ... When I go out I want to have fun, so it's in a gay club ... That's it. I'm very closed-minded [*laughing*] ... in that way. So I'd be easy to reach as a bisexual. Even if I'm in a straight relationship, I got all gay friends. I like to hang out in gay organizations, gay clubs ... So I think bisexual people who are like me would be easy to reach in that way, but that would be kind of the easy way to go about it ... We'd have to find a place where bisexual people no matter where they live or what their background is ... they have to go there one time or another ... like a hospital ... like all the hospitals, all the CLSCs ... places like that would maybe be something general and neutral where bisexual people would just stumble onto the information ... But if ... if other bisexual people are not like me, they wouldn't be so easy to reach.

Our data suggest that effective HIV education with people who have sexual relations with both men and women, then, needs to situate itself outside an identity-based logic. Rather than naming bisexuality, or situating bisexuals as a subpopulation within gay and lesbian communities, prevention needs to locate itself in very mainstream settings. Information and services are to be delivered not by a specialized HIV/AIDS organization (such as one dedicated to the needs of gay men), but are to be integrated in general sexual health care for everyday people.

The desire to have mainstream HIV/STD prevention materials extended to the overall tenor of a campaign. As we observed in chapters 4 and 5, participants wanted to see a full diversity of people represented, in gender, age, and culture. Relatedly, they contend that current HIV education is too similar to other kinds of marketing in society. Two interviewees comment on current educational materials we showed them:

A top-down kind of thing with an ad campaign like this. It seems to me it was run by rich people. This was a campaign that was conceived by rich people, who hired somebody else. Nobody is HIV-positive in this whole crew, from the artistic designer to … And especially not the people who hired them, who came up with the concept in the first place: they don't have AIDS, they're not HIV-positive.

It's good to remind people that AIDS is still around, because I think a lot of people think that it's not, which is really not good at all. But it's too market*y*. You know what I mean? Like, it seems it was put together by people who could do advertising.

The reservations expressed about these advertisements are related, in part, to their content – for instance, how a poster with bed headboards as tombstones reinforces an equation between HIV and death, and how such a message can increase the stigma of HIV-positive people. But these quotations also raise critical questions about the overall orientation and packaging of such materials. They situate it as just another marketing ploy, in a world already saturated with consumer marketing techniques. A more effective strategy identified by our participants would be to orient education in a more 'regular' manner – with 'normal' bodies and people represented, devoid of the usual publicity hype. People wanted a more simple, community-based approach to education.

Our interviewees offer suggestions about concrete ways to facilitate access to information about sexual health. Enthusiastic about a mainstream approach to education and services, the people with whom we spoke offered some useful ideas on how to orient prevention materials, as well as how to deliver services. Distribution of materials in everyday venues, an approach that does not privilege identity, a framework outside more common marketing, and a discreet orientation were cited as useful strategies for HIV prevention in a manner relevant to people who have sexual relations with both men and women. Furthermore, there is a need to link education to services directly, since people often search out information about sexual health when they need such specific services.

Conclusion

In this chapter, we have examined the problems bisexuals experience accessing relevant information about HIV and STDs. One of the most important findings of our research is that the provision of information must be linked to good health services as well, so that people have a clear place to go if and when they have questions. Yet to consider health services for bisexuals and swingers raises a host of other issues, since there are major obstacles to accessing such services. Our research here has considered what some of these main barriers are, in addition to providing concrete recommendations for change. This nexus of education/ services is a fundamental backdrop to think about how to engage in HIV prevention more effectively. While the data are specific to individuals who are sexually involved with both sexes, they also provide a way to think about organizing HIV/STD information and services differently for all kinds of people.

This chapter contains a wealth of empirical data on the difficulties people have finding the information they need. Yet it goes further than noting that such problems exist. Indeed, our research demonstrates that one reason people who have sexual relations with both men and women cannot get good information about their sexual health is that they have poor access to (sexual) health services. Misconceptions and ignorance of bisexuality, lack of access to condoms for swingers, and the dismissal of bisexual women's specific health needs are the more salient issues identified in this regard. As the participants make clear throughout this chapter, access to health services structures the kinds of information people can or cannot have, as well as how this information can inform their actions. This situation is in turn linked to the particular knowledge we have of HIV/ AIDS: an invocation of scientific knowledge in which women are not at risk of STDs makes it difficult (if not impossible in certain instances) to offer services that address women's needs. Knowledge informs services, which in turn affect the type and kind of information available.

This insight is significant for our broader project, for helping us to understand how and why there are no HIV prevention materials in Canada specifically adapted to men and women with bisexual behaviour, more than twenty-five years into an epidemic. A lack of education for these people reflects a broader social relation in which they are neglected within sexual health services. The suggestions put forward by participants offer preliminary strategies to intervene in this situation. They contend that the challenge is greater than simply creating prevention materials with relevant information for bisexuals. While the specific content of education certainly needs to be adapted to the complex and multiple realities discussed above, it must also be distributed in and through relevant health agencies. Education cannot be divorced from services.

While our data provide clear indication of the need to link education to services, it is noteworthy in this discussion just how difficult it can be to engage in such initiatives – challenges that in certain instances arise from the administrative apparatus of funding HIV education. Let us return to the Specific Populations Fund discussed in chapter 2. As we have seen, the program exists to support projects that engage in HIV prevention with particular communities. The fund is further subdivided into three priorities: the first clearly focuses on prevention for affected populations; the second addresses stigma and discrimination related to HIV and AIDS; and the third is concerned with training service providers and increasing the capacity of people who work within community-based AIDS service organizations and health care institutions.[4] Taken together, these three elements of the fund are said to offer a comprehensive response to HIV/AIDS prevention in particular communities identified in the fund.

Yet careful reflection on the different priorities reveals that education and services have been segregated within this initiative. Applications are required to address one of the three priorities of the fund. One can prepare a grant application concerned with the development and distribution of prevention materials (priority one). Alternatively, one can develop a project that focuses on training health care and social service providers on a specific aspect of HIV/AIDS, and or a particular way of working with people who use services (priority three). But one cannot, at least not in any simple sense, outline a project that deals simultaneously with prevention and education. Funding for programs within the Specific Populations Fund are targeted to prevention *or* services, not to a critical nexus between them.

This way of thinking about responding to HIV/AIDS, of course, stands at odds with the data presented throughout this chapter. Yet it is important to consider, because as we argue in chapter 2, the administration of HIV/AIDS funding determines the shape of specific programs, the daily work that community organizations do, and the recognition of the people whom such agencies serve – as well as those whom are overlooked. The voices of participants tell us of the importance of linking education to services. At the same time, our analysis of HIV/AIDS funding here considers the extent to which state support of HIV/AIDS work requires a tidy separation between education and services. Current HIV education is divorced from services in part because the funding of programs itself requires such a division. Such an administrative structure is at odds with recent critical research that demonstrates the importance of integrating HIV prevention and treatment in our response to the epidemic (Mykalovskiy et al. 2009).

The voices of participants cited here, then, are useful – indispensable, actually – to a nuanced understanding of how to engage in HIV prevention more effectively. Participants recount their need to access sexual health information and sexual health services at the same time. Moreover, with specific regard to sexual health services, the men and women we interviewed describe numerous experiences in which they were misunderstood, neglected, and/or dismissed, and in which they lack access to primary prevention materials and information. These dealings with health services certainly point to the need for training of health care and social service providers working in this field, and the people cited have offered useful starting points for developing services that are relevant for them.

The experiences outlined by participants document the line of fault between what they need (an education/services nexus, and decent access to services free of discrimination) and what is available (information that is not adapted to their lives, poor access to health care services, and disregard for their specific needs). The interviews yield insight, then, into how the gaps of current HIV/AIDS work are actually created by organizing our knowledge of the epidemic in a particular way. By beginning with this kind of analysis, one focused on knowledge itself, we can offer a critical reading of the bureaucratic infrastructure of HIV/AIDS funding. In this manner, attention to the voices of everyday people can assist us in better understanding how health care is administered, as well as the ways that exclusion of people can be organized in it.

Of course, to have such a nuanced understanding of how exclusion is structured within institutions, as well as its impact, is significant. Yet is it sufficient merely to provide an analysis of how this functions? Is it enough simply to document the exclusion of people with partners of both sexes from HIV education and services? Indeed, if we have detailed knowledge of how and why this particular type of exclusion persists, what can be done about it? The next chapter addresses this challenge, exploring the specific actions we developed that would link the knowledge we had gathered to concrete action in the social and institutional world.

7 Connecting Knowledge and Action: Development and Distribution of HIV and STD Prevention Materials

Contentons-nous de faire réfléchir, n'essayons pas de convaincre.

– Georges Braque

Drawing on the tradition of participatory action research, we sought to integrate concrete intervention into the problems that the people we interviewed experience accessing information and services. As researchers, but also as activists, we wanted our work to be able to offer something – to be more than a simple documentation of these problems, more than a report that sits on a shelf. From the initial conception of this project, then, we envisioned an action component, specifically in the development of appropriate educational materials. Beginning with the needs articulated by our participants, we wanted to use our data to develop the kinds of prevention they said was desired. In this manner, action was not just something that could hypothetically emerge from the research results. Rather, the action component of the research is integral to the project and not to be separated from its epistemological and methodological orientations (Stringer 1999). Moreover, this particular understanding of the connection between knowledge and action embodies the community-based research principle of *relevance*, outlined in chapter 3. The educational materials to be developed are designed to fill gaps in the existing prevention, notably in responding to the issues identified as important by our interviewees. In this chapter, we discuss different ways in which our project works at both research and action – at gathering empirical data and setting them into motion. The primary manner in which this was achieved was by developing specific educational posters. Yet our work also involved some action components throughout the research process. In the next section, we turn our attention to the ways in which we sought to intervene in the current situation even before we developed specific posters.

Actions during the Research Process

Our conceptualization of this project involved first studying what people who have sexual relations with both men and women would like to have in HIV and STD prevention information, and then working to translate these findings into appropriate materials. Within such a model, inquiry informs action. Yet the process of doing this research raised methodological and ethical questions that interrogate such a model. In certain instances, the research process itself reveals the need for immediate action. Three specific elements of our data underline this dynamic.

The first situation has already been discussed. In our interviews with the managers and owners of swinger establishments in Montréal, they noted that they did not have access to inexpensive and/or free condoms. Moreover, they wondered if we could possibly assist in this regard. As academic researchers, we could have replied that our final report would note this absence, and make a recommendation that public health provide specific outreach to swinger communities and facilitate access to primary prevention materials. While of course necessary, such an approach would not improve the situation in the short term – at best, it would promise to describe the current gaps, with a hypothetical improvement to come at some unspecified time. We proceeded differently and contacted a local community-based HIV/AIDS organization and asked them to supply condoms and lubricant to the particular establishment in question. Such a strategy sought to offer assistance immediately. While undoubtedly incomplete (the supply of condoms was only to one establishment and ignored the many other swinger businesses and private parties in Montréal), nonetheless it illustrates the specific action we took to help improve the current situation.

The second anecdote we recount in this regard is similar and has also been presented. A workshop on safer sex and contraception, organized by the local group Bi Unité Montréal (BUM), invited a local HIV/AIDS organization to provide the training. Yet as we have seen in chapter 6, the content and orientation of this workshop ignored women entirely. If we regard this situation as researchers, it offers compelling evidence of the ways in which HIV/AIDS information and services are implicitly gendered. In this regard, the workshop is part of the general data to support our argument that there are serious gaps in the delivery of education and services. But if we consider the situation from the perspective of the men and women present, its urgency requires an attitude more engaged than simply collecting data. Women in particular did not have the information they needed to protect themselves – and they went to the workshop, of course, with the objective of seeking out such information! Since we work in this specific area, we were in a unique position to be offer such information. Following the workshop, we sent pertinent education about woman-to-woman transmission of HIV and STDs to BUM, who in turn distributed it to the association's members. Here again, we facilitated access to relevant HIV/STD materials for the men and women we interviewed in the short term.

The central concern of our research project – access to information – requires critical reflection on our ethical relations with project participants. Indeed, we wanted to speak to people about the kind of information they needed. Yet on the basis of our review of the scientific studies, as well as our knowledge of bisexual realities, we hypothesized that most people who have sexual relations with both men and women would not have the information they needed to protect themselves against HIV and STD transmission. If we as researchers and activists had such information within our reach, should we not – from an ethical perspective – provide it to our participants? Is it morally acceptable to conduct research that documents gaps in information but does not provide the type of information needed when it is available? How can one balance the needs of participants (to access information adapted to their needs) with the needs of research (to collect data on a particular problematic)?

In thinking about these questions, we developed a strategy that would, we hoped, satisfy both the scientific requirements of good research (the collection of data) as well as the ethical matters bound within conducting our project (giving people the information they need). For each interview, we prepared a resource package. The package contained pertinent information on HIV/AIDS – everything from a general overview, to transmission of HIV and STDs between women. We also included contact information for specific services, so that people would be able to continue to inform themselves once the interview was over. The interview itself asked people about their gaps in information, including whether or not they had specific questions. However, we did not immediately answer such questions for participants.

Such a strategy could transform the interview entirely, from one in which we asked participants to tell us their knowledge, to one in which we offered services. Rather, during the interview interviewers would note specific questions and state that we would return to these matters. Once the interview reached a conclusion, we would offer participants the resource package. In so doing, we would often return to the specific technical questions that respondents may have raised, as in the following example:

> Q : Bon alors je vais te donner la trousse de, des infos. Tu as mentionné … alors on a comme des ressources, ben sur des groupes bisexuels à Montréal.
> R : Oui.
> Q : Pis aussi euh sur dépistage, ligne d'écoute, des choses comme ça.
> R : Mais c'est intéressant ça.
> Q : Oui. Pis ça c'est tout un … comme un … des questions que tu peux avoir. Pis il a des choses je pense spécifiques euh sur euh … entre femmes.
> R : OK.
> Q : Parce que je pense que c'est ça que tu as mentionné.
> R : Oui.
> Q : Alors là c'est un peu où on est rendu avec … parce que je sais que c'est toujours une question et que c'est pas clair.
> R : Moi, je vais lire ça tout de suite après là.
>
> (Q: Good, so now I'm going to give you a resource package. You mentioned … so there are resources, bisexual groups in Montréal.
> R: Yes.
> Q: Oh, and also on testing, an information line, things like that.
> A: Oh, that's interesting.
> Q: Yes. That's it, it's all, like, the questions you could have. And there are things I think specific on … between women.
> R: OK.
> Q: Because I think you mentioned that.
> R: Yes.
> Q: So that's about what we have, because I know it's always a question and it's not always clear.
> R: I'm going to read this right away.)

By offering people access to the information they needed, we hoped that our research embodied an ethical commitment to our responsibilities towards participants. At the same time, we offered this information at the end of the session, to ensure that the interview itself fulfilled an objective of collecting new data and evidence.

Participants were especially appreciative of this information, as well as the fact that the resource package included contact details for relevant services:

Q : C'est ça que je te disais tout à l'heure.
R : Hm-hm.
Q : Toutes les affaires de même, toi tu les, tu les as là sur un papier, tu nous les donnes.
R : Oui.
Q : C'est ça que je te dis, on peut les avoir ces affaires-là, mais juste par les organismes.
R : Oui.
Q : Des gens comme vous autres tu sais, qui fait des recherches ou ben euh … tu sais ils … comment je peux dire ça? T'en trouves pas partout de ça … Tu sais, si tu sais pas où t'en procurer, tu en auras jamais … Regarde, vous autres vous en donnez là … Mais je le savais même pas que vous en aviez ici … Mais s'il y aurait des affaires expliquées, comme genre où se procurer ce papier-là, des renseignements, des … des places qui seraient plus vites … Le monde il serait plus intéressé … c'est ça que je te disais tout à l'heure quand je disais, c'est ben beau des pamphlets pis des affaires, mais si tu le sais pas où tu les procurer.

(Q: That's what I was saying to you just now.
R: Hm-hm.
Q: All those things, you have, you have them on paper, you give us that.
R: Yes.
Q: That's what I'm saying, we can get those kinds of things, but just through organizations.
R: People like you, who do research, you know, how do I say this? You don't find them just anywhere. You know, if you don't know where to get this, you'll never get it. Look, you give it. But I didn't even know that you would have it here. If there would be explicit things, like how to get this paper, information, places where it would be quicker, people would be more interested. That's what I was saying earlier when I say, pamphlets are all well and good and things like that, but if you don't know how to get them.)

Well, I am glad that you offer some resources. Like, since we're going through it, I think it's good to throw that in at the end, too.

The distribution of such resource packages thus represented a specific form of action, at the level of contact with individual participants. The action component of this approach did not go unnoticed:

> Ben je trouve ça bien que vous complétez l'entrevue avec de l'information supplémentaire ... Ça peut être important et euh ... pis intéressant aussi hein ... Pour explorer d'autres euh ... ça j'imagine que ça fait partie d'une autre genre de campagne de sensibilisation?

> (Well, I think it's good that you end the interview with supplementary information. That can be important, interesting too, to explore other ... I imagine that's part of another education campaign?)

As this participant underlines, by providing people with information adapted to their specific needs, our research intervenes in the current gaps in HIV education and services. In this manner, our work integrated an action component into every interview.

Building on such elements of action, our project sought to consider the empirical data with the objective of developing educational materials. The next section of this chapter examines how we went about this work, as well as how the prevention materials respond to the major concerns in accessing information and services identified by our participants.

Development of Educational Posters

Participants had identified a variety of formats for HIV education, from radio advertisements to materials distributed in the Publi-Sac. The research team and Advisory Committee considered the different possibilities offered in order to think about what format would best reach people who have sexual relations with both men and women. The idea of posters was repeatedly raised and promised to be effective, provided that they were distributed in mainstream locations. Although the other suggestions are certainly worth pursuing, we limited our creation to posters in order to narrow our focus. Moreover, some of the suggestions offered were beyond the reach of our budget (here, we too are constrained by our institutional locations and funding arrangements): however exciting it would be to create a movie trailer for distribution in movie theatres, or to develop an educational hot air balloon in the shape of a condom, our budget for the development and distribution of materials did not permit such initiatives.

How, then, did we go about creating relevant educational materials? As outlined in chapter 3 on methodology, we organized our data collection in relation to three different 'networks' of people who have sexual relations with both men and women: bisexual women, swingers, and people who are sexually involved with both men and women but without necessarily naming themselves 'bisexual.' Our recruitment and data collection took place in that order: we interviewed approximately thirty individuals in each 'network.' The posters that we developed, then, reflect some of the specific realities situated within these three networks.

The first set of data that we examined, then, was specific to bisexual women. As we have argued in chapters 5 and 6 in particular, women do not have access to basic prevention information about HIV and STDs. Our challenge was to create a poster that could provide such information. In examining our data, however, and in considering the scientific issues at stake (the actual transmission of STDs and HIV between women), we were rather challenged as to what specific content could be placed on a poster. What could we say to women that was relevant, not fear-based, of practical import, and linked to services? Should we focus on a particular STD – say, the transmission of trichomoniasis between women – or should we offer a broader perspective on sexual health? What should we say – if anything – about dental dams? And how could we possibly fit everything we needed to say on one poster? Although we had interviewed a large group of women about their needs, and although we certainly had a wealth of empirical data upon which to draw, the process of creating educational materials began with more questions than answers.

The more we talked – about what the women wanted, but also about the complexity of the issues involved in creating relevant prevention that addresses transmission between women – the more we realized that there was, in fact, no escaping the reality that there are more questions that answers. Returning to our data from the interviews, we considered this issue with regards to the approach that is usually taken in HIV education. Our participants told us that prevention materials try to send a message about what one can do that is frequently summarized by the ideas 'Use a condom,' 'Protect yourself,' or, 'If you do not use a condom you will contract HIV and die.' In this regard, public health education establishes itself as a requisite authority and tells people what to do in their sexual behaviour. We have already considered the ways in which people disregard such a message, and part of the rejection of such education is because, as one interviewee notes, it is a very top-down approach. Moreover, it is difficult to imagine developing a similar approach on the subject of woman-to-woman transmission of HIV. While there are documented cases of such transmission, one cannot deny that the risk is lesser than in the case of unprotected anal relations between men. All of these dilemmas then led us to think about orienting our posters differently. Rather than trying to send a message that tells people what to do, based on our expert knowledge (for example, a poster that encourages women to use dental dams for oral sex and gloves for vaginal fisting), we decided to begin with the notion of questions. Indeed, if the women we interviewed had questions about these issues, and if the answers are complex indeed (we elaborate below on our position on the use of dental dams), then a framework that acknowledges such questions and complexities is warranted. Furthermore, orienting our education in such a manner would avoid a top-down approach and underline the fact that it is perfectly acceptable to have questions about how HIV and STDs are transmitted. If our posters include contact information for a website and a telephone number, they would also link education to services. In this manner, the objective of the poster is not to tell women what to do. Rather, by asking a question and pointing the way to obtain more information, we wanted this poster to help hook women up to appropriate health services.

Examining our data, we quickly realized that it would be difficult – if not impossible – to develop even a poster that satisfies everyone. Some participants wanted us to include multiple partners, while others warned against representing threesomes and reinforcing clichés of bisexuals as sexually promiscuous. As we went about creating education, we quickly realized that *one* poster would be insufficient. We decided to develop a number of different posters, then, whose visual imagery would include a diversity of women (in age, physical beauty according to cultural norms, ethnocultural communities) and a variety of sexual realities (multiple partners, stable relationship with another woman).

Our different 'kinds' of posters would target different women – for example, we elected to include one specific to older women, and one that addressed a younger female audience.

The text accompanying the posters was narrowed down to two slogans. (Here again, we felt that one text could not possibly satisfy participants' different demands.) Both slogans are located within the general framework of asking questions outlined above. One reads, 'Je sais quoi faire pour me protéger avec un homme. Mais avec une femme?' (I know what safer sex is with him. But with her?). The second text reads, 'Ma blonde ma dit qu'on ne peut pas attraper de maladies entre femmes. Mon chum, lui, le sait pas. Pis toi?' (My girlfriend says you can't get an STD from a woman. My boyfriend is clueless about these things. What do you think?) Within the latter example, the question is expressed in an extremely informal, colloquial manner ('Pis toi?'). This strategy is one that uses everyday language to provide education. Moreover, it is resolutely and typically Québécois. Both in semantics and in tone, one could not imagine a similar use of language within a health promotion advertisement produced in France, for example, where social relations are more formal and codified.

The visual images that we created to accompany these texts were varied. One series of images is of an animation type. Different types and ages of women are pictured in order to represent diversity among women (see figures 7.1 to 7.6). A second advertisement targets older women (figure 7.7), while a third poster is directed towards a younger audience (figure 7.8). We also developed a fourth advertisement in which the facial expression of the model indicates someone who is asking a question (figure 7.9).

In choice of photographic models, we wanted to ensure that the overall tone of the posters maintained a 'community-based' feel, in keeping with the needs articulated by the women we interviewed. As such, rather than hiring professional models through an agency (an option that was, in any event, beyond our budget!), we placed a classified advertisement in a free weekly paper asking for interested women to submit their photos for consideration to participate in our educational campaign. We selected the women to be photographed on the basis of our discussions in the Advisory Committee of our different visual needs. To our pleasant surprise, the women expressed enthusiasm for participating in the campaign, even though the honorarium we were able to offer was essentially symbolic.

Once we had organized a photo shoot and had taken many different pictures of the women, we narrowed down the images to be chosen in conjunction with the slogans discussed above. The final results of this process – which itself took several months, from the time we advertised for models to holding the photo shoot and selecting final images – resulted in the creation of several different HIV/STD posters targeted to women who have sexual relations with both women and men (see figures 7.7 to 7.9).

Figure 7.1

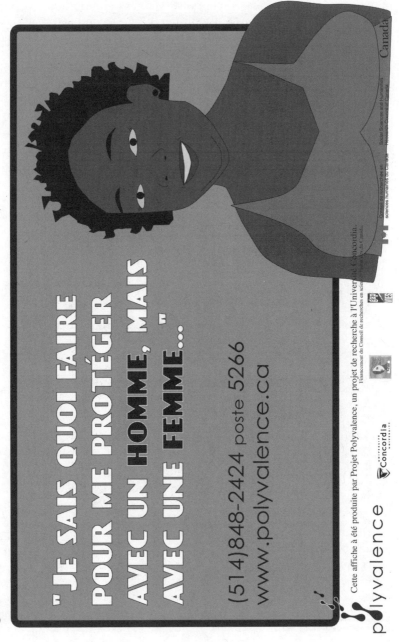

Figure 7.2

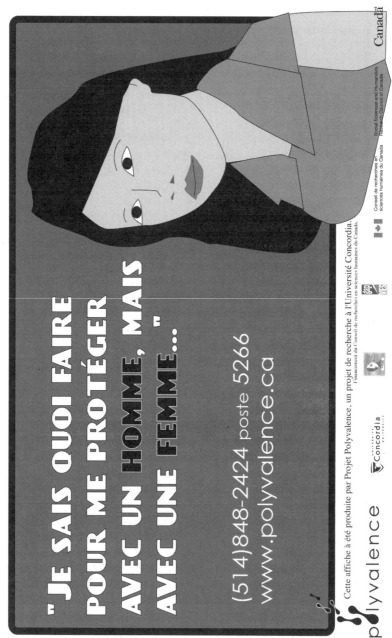

Figure 7.3

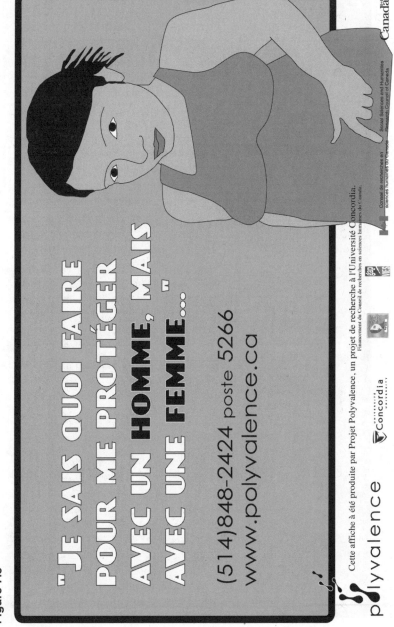

Figure 7.4

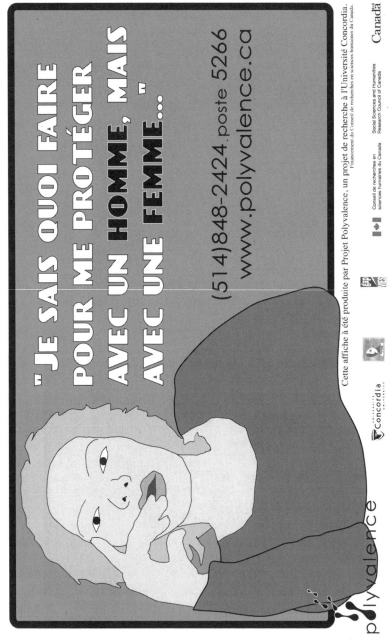

Figure 7.5

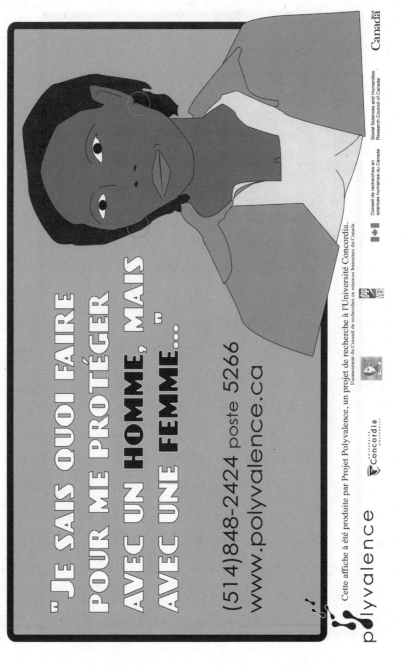

Figure 7.6

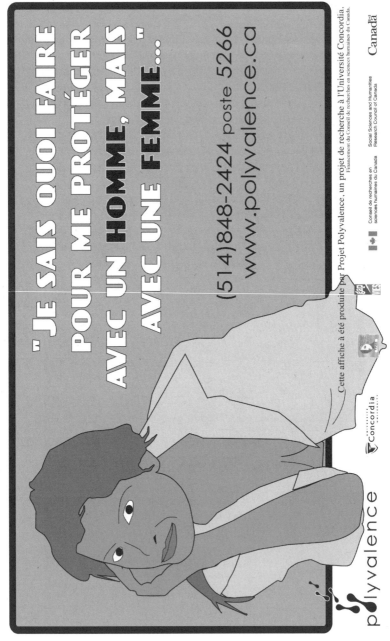

Figure 7.7

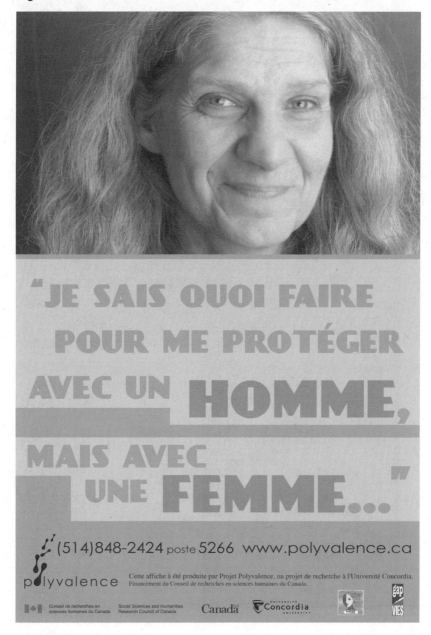

Figure 7.8

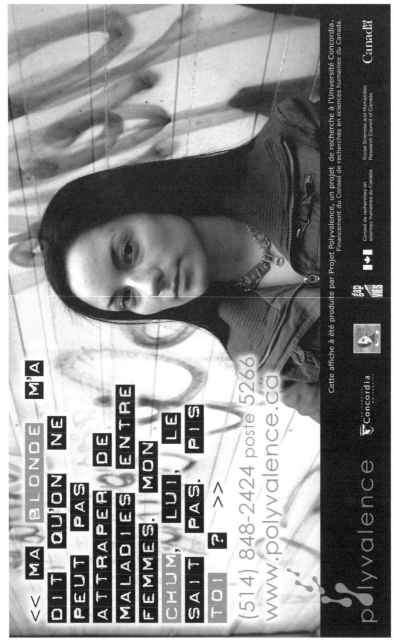

Figure 7.9

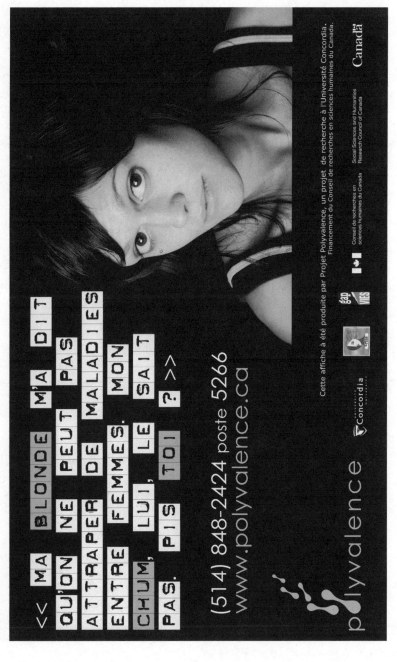

The data we collected indicated that people wanted educational posters to include both a telephone number of an HIV/STD information service and a website address. Both of these tactics, according to our interviewees, would link prevention education to sexual health services. With regards to an HIV/STD information line, we collaborated with CRISS – le Centre de ressources et d'interventions sur la santé et la sexualité, a community-based organization dedicated to HIV and STD prevention and services in Montréal, who operate a free telephone information line. By having their information line on our posters, we would immediately facilitate access to information, as well as services. (We would, however, provide training on matters specific to bisexuality so as to ensure that people who answered the phone were knowledgeable about specific issues and resources.)

If collaboration with an existing community organization and information line was relatively simple to ensure access to information and services for people who would choose to call for resources, the question of information to be put on a website was more challenging. Indeed, having reviewed the needs of participants, as well as available information that we could find online, we confronted difficulty. There was not, in our opinion, a website that already existed that had the kind of information required – especially information about the transmission of HIV and STDs between women. We could locate various educational projects and initiatives from around the world[1] and certainly take some inspiration from them, but we could not find the specific information adapted and relevant for women in an existing website – particularly written in French. Moreover, since our data analysis indicates the need to link prevention to services, it was apparent to us that any website listed on a poster would need to include relevant resources for health services in Montréal. Having considered these complex issues, then, we decided that our project needed to create its own website for inclusion on posters (see www.polyvalence.ca). Here, we could group the relevant information (including links to other projects around the world that might be of interest), as well as local sexual health services in Montréal. This development emerged out of the research itself: it was not something that we had imagined (or predicted in our budget) when we submitted the grant proposal. Nevertheless, since we wanted to create educational materials that were relevant, and information about prevention and services adapted to our participants was required, the development of our project website was a necessity. This situation reveals some of the particular challenges faced in action research: if a research project makes a commitment to action at the outset (as ours did, having included an objective of providing relevant education to men and women with bisexual sexual practices), the follow-through of the research can be labour-intensive indeed. We were faced with the challenge of developing a specific website that would have relevant information and services – no small undertaking. Such a challenge suggests one of the reasons why action research is not always popular within university-based scholarship (Stringer 1999): to document problems in accessing information is one matter, to act on them is another one entirely.

The specific content of the website was determined in relation to our data analysis (see www.polyvalence.ca). We offer basic information about transmission of HIV/AIDS, as well as details specific to transmission between women and information adapted to swingers (the importance of changing condoms). We also include relevant information about STD transmission, with links to the modes of transmission, symptoms, and treatment of different infections. A specific section of our website is dedicated to condoms – basic information on their use, as well as where one can obtain free condoms in Montréal. With regards to services, our website contains resources for bisexuals and swingers – from community associations to local clubs and saunas. We offer links to some educational materials adapted to people who have sexual relations with both men and women – materials created elsewhere, notably in France, Germany, and the United States. Furthermore, we include information on accessing health services more generally – HIV tests, general STD check-ups, vaccination against hepatitis A and B, and gynaecological resources. Since the project emerges from research, we reproduce a summary of the study, as well as the main recommendations. We also present a section of the website on community-based research, so that people can find more information about this particular kind of research practice. Finally, our website contains images of the different posters and educational materials that we created. In all of these ways, our website seeks to provide exactly the kind of information that the people we interviewed require: whether that be specific technical details on the transmission of herpes, names of relevant associations and community resources, or contact information for some sexual health services themselves.

One specific element of the website content deserves particular analysis here: the information on woman-to-woman transmission of HIV. As we outlined earlier, there are documented cases of such transmission.

That said, the risks are not as high as unprotected vaginal or anal sex. Yet when it comes to specific educational materials developed to address this matter, one notes a curious contradiction. Either woman-to-woman transmission of HIV and STDs is ignored entirely (this is usually the case), or else the presentation of the information insists that women must use dental dams and latex gloves in their sexual relations with other women. Furthermore, as Robin Gorna maintains, the latter kind of information is rather specific to the United States, when it is available.

Like Gorna, we decided to address the matter of woman-to-woman transmission from a perspective different from that advocated in the United States. To be sure, we acknowledge that there is risk of HIV transmission between women and that the transmission of other STDs between women is even more remarkable. That said, we also acknowledge that few women use dental dams and latex gloves when with other women, and rates of HIV transmission between women remain low in comparison to other groups. We approach this issue, then, from the perspective of risk reduction. If a woman is interested in ensuring that there is zero risk of HIV transmission between women, then indeed the use of dental dams and latex gloves is warranted. If, however, a woman is prepared to accept a low risk of transmission, then she can make an informed decision to forego the use of such materials. This kind of approach – while certainly at odds with that favoured in the United States (Gorna 1996) – is similar to recommendations for oral sex performed on a man, in which oral sex without a condom is considered to be a low-risk (but not a zero-risk) activity. To frame the matter of woman-to-woman transmission in this way is to move beyond the 'all-or-nothing' approach historically available, in which either women have to use latex all the time, or else no specific mention of woman-to-woman transmission is available. Furthermore, the information we include encourages women to evaluate the level of risk they are prepared to accept and conduct themselves accordingly. Interestingly, we could not find HIV education on woman-to-woman transmission that adopts a risk-reduction framework – an absence in marked contrast to HIV education directed to gay men that appeals to risk reduction as a viable strategy. We had to then write the text for what such an approach could look like when speaking about woman-to-woman transmission, as we could not find it elsewhere.

The first set of interviews we conducted, then, resulted in both the creation of specific educational materials, and the development of a project website. These actions were complemented by the development of posters for the two other networks of people we interviewed: swingers and people who have sexual relations with both men and women.

With specific regard to swingers, the process of creating our posters again began with the data analysis. We considered the gaps in existing information, what people wanted to see, as well as how to package and orient the materials. On the last subject, we took inspiration from the words of one participant in particular who suggested how to frame an advertisement:

Mais il faudrait que, vraiment qu'il y ait deux couples dessus. Un couple à gauche, un couple à droite ... Pour vraiment euh dire ... même pas de mentionner échangistes, juste de voir les deux couples. Euh on saurait tout de suite que c'est deux couples qui sont échangistes, tout simplement ... Je trouve que ce serait ou un couple avec une femme ou avec un homme ... Là ce serait vraiment euh ... t'aurais même pas, la, juste la photo parlerait. Sauf que quand même il faudrait que tu spécifierais plus euh ... du côté euh ... les MTS ou ben sur le côté VIH. Mais pas vraiment beaucoup. Juste des petites notes de rien. Mais juste la photo parlerait.

(But you'd need really two couples on it. One couple on the left, one on the right. To really say ... not even to mention swingers, just to see two couples. We would simply know right away that it's two couples who are swingers. I think that it would be either a couple with a woman or with a man. That would be really ... you wouldn't even have ... just the photo would speak. But you'd have to specify, all the same, more about STDs or HIV. But not really a lot. Just little notes. Just the photo would speak.)

The concept we developed to embody such an approach was that of four people in a hot tub (see figure 7.10). The idea of a hot tub appeals to a certain cliché of swinger culture, and we relied on it to signify the context. As before, we placed classified advertisement to find our models, so as to ensure everyday people are represented. Like the previous advertisements discussed, we begin with the notion of questions. The text reads, 'Questions sur votre santé sexuelle?' (Questions about your sexual health?) The point is not to tell people what to do didactically. Rather, we encourage people to ask questions about their sexual health. By including a website address and telephone number, we provide concrete ways to find more information, as well as to access sexual health services.

In the final poster we developed, we wanted to address relations with both men and women, but very implicitly. For this advertisement in particular, we wanted to deliberately steer clear of explicit references to bisexuality or sexual orientation. The concept we developed was two-fold: a sexual scenario between two men and a woman was represented in the background, while the foreground of the poster contains a close-up of an individual's calendar / day planner (see figure 7.11). The specific information on the calendar reflects details of everyday life – a date to get one's hair cut, or an appointment with a veterinarian. Moreover, the calendar includes some references specific to an active sexual life – a 'siesta' on a Saturday afternoon with a woman, a dinner with a man with the reminder, 'Get the champagne.' One specific date is also marked, and circled in red to stand out, with the phrase, 'Find an STD clinic.' In keeping with our research results, we use the term *STD* and not *STI* (sexually transmitted infection), because our primary objective is to have people understand our message, and we need to employ the language with which they are familiar. The information on the calendar provides an implicit reference to bisexuality, as does the visual image in the background. The specific entry 'Find an STD clinic' encourages people to locate and access relevant sexual health services – an important part of having an active sexual life. This poster, then, offers HIV education within a much broader context of sexual health.

The posters that we developed make a concerted effort to offer the kind of prevention desired by the men and women we interviewed: information relevant to their sexualities and lives; recognition of multiple partners and specific prevention issues; a mainstream approach; avoidance of an identity-based logic; the provision of practical information; the inclusion of a diversity of people in age, gender, culture, and physical body type; use of plain language; and a strategy that links education to health services. Taken together, the different posters appeal to different realities: some are oriented towards older women, while others are more specifically for swingers. Some posters include multiple partners, while others acknowledge such a reality as merely one possibility among others. In all of these ways, the different posters represent an effort to create and offer the type of HIV and STD prevention materials identified as necessary by our participants.

The creation of these different posters was a necessary first step to act on the current situation. However, we needed to do more than to develop prevention materials; we also needed to distribute them in the public sphere. Having reserved some money from our budget in this

Figure 7.10

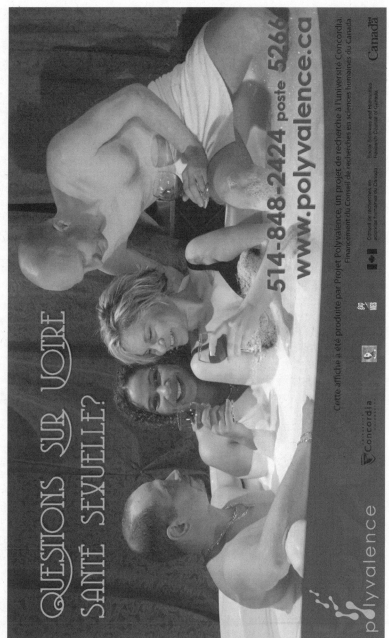

Figure 7.11

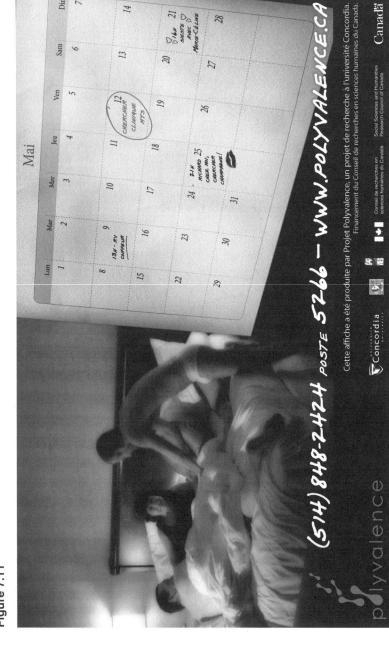

regard (we had made provisions for this in our research funding proposal), we organized a small-scale educational campaign. Using four of
the posters that we developed, we reproduced the materials within free
weekly newspapers in Montréal for one month. While developing the
posters, we had collaborated with the community organization CRISS
to use the phone number of their HIV/STD information line. However,
the organization dissolved by the time we were ready to implement
our educational campaign, so we were without a telephone number to
include on the posters. Since there was no other free HIV or STD information line Québec at the time, we decided to organize our own telephone
line for the duration of our campaign. While labour-intensive, this strategy ensured that the people responding to the line were well trained
in the needs expressed by our participants.[2] In addition to our posters,
we had an information booth at Salon de l'Amour et de la séduction,
a large-scale trade fair related to sex and sexuality in Montréal. There,
we reproduced a much broader cross-section of our posters (blown up
to a large scale), and distributed over two thousand postcards with the
image from our 'swinger' advertisement (see figure 7.10). We also organized a party to promote the results of our research.

Our campaign was largely successful in reaching the people we targeted. Within the month we conducted the campaign, our website had
2113 visits, 1801 of which were new visitors. The average time spent
on our site was three minutes, 42 seconds, and the different pages
and submenus of our website were consulted in the following order
of frequency: bisexual (728 visits), swingers (628 visits), HIV (508 visits), STDs (356 visits), condoms (215 visits), and links (209 visits). The
telephone information line received on average from three to ten calls
per day. Some callers requested more information about the party we
were organizing, while others had specific questions about HIV and
STD transmission. Given that this was an entirely new health promotion project with limited resources for publicity, we felt that such a
response was positive indeed (both in website visits and information
calls). We did get the word out about our project and helped people
obtain access to information and services with regard to their sexual
health, but we were less successful with the organization of our party:
few people attended, despite the wide publicity. Given that many of
us had previously organized such parties in the past, we remain somewhat perplexed about the poor attendance: perhaps it was due to the
choice of venue or the specific location in the city. Nevertheless, we
remain satisfied that many people in Montréal were exposed to our

educational materials and that they took some additional steps to find out more about this initiative (whether by consulting our website or calling our information line).

Conclusion

This chapter considers the ways in which our research connects knowledge and action. During the research process itself, we provided participants with the information they require about HIV and STD transmission and facilitated access to primary prevention materials for one swinger establishment in particular. Moreover, our project developed specific educational posters that would have the content and orientation cited as necessary by our participants to be effective. To be sure, these posters do not offer any kind of magical solution. Yet given the absence of prevention materials specific to bisexual men and women, they offer a useful point of departure. Perhaps most importantly, they underline the fact that it is possible to engage in critical research that does more than offer a commentary on a situation. By linking the design and distribution of these materials to our empirical data, we demonstrate the contribution that an action research framework can make to both scientific knowledge and community education.

Conclusion

This book project offers a consideration of the absence of HIV prevention materials for people who have sexual relations with both men and
women. As we have seen, in order to understand why there is so little
education specific to bisexual men and women, we need to think about
interlocking elements of HIV work. We began our inquiry with epistemological questions, in an effort to unpack how we know what we
know about sexuality and HIV. Here, we demonstrated the manner
in which our conceptual frames of sexuality make bisexuality literally
impossible. These questions of knowledge are closely linked to methods and methodology, which is to say with how we go about gathering data. Our analysis of epidemiology considers the manner in which
scientific investigations are limited in a number of respects: from making bisexuals disappear, to minimizing women's vulnerabilities to HIV
transmission, to reinforcing certain cultural stereotypes of race and
sexuality. In all of these ways, our work demonstrates how scientific
research is informed by, and embedded within, broader social relations.

Having analysed these epistemological and methodological dilemmas, we go on to examine how HIV education is organized, institutionally speaking. Decisions about what kinds of communities warrant
attention, and why, are both implicit and explicit within a bureaucratic
infrastructure that manages the HIV/AIDS epidemic and our collective response to it. Drawing on the framework known as institutional
ethnography, we reflect on the manner in which HIV policy neglects
bisexual realities, and how it (ironically) does so at the precise moment
bisexual men are scapegoated as vectors of transmission for heterosexual women. Close readings of central policy documents and funding
initiatives allow us to consider how and why individuals who have

sexual relations with both men and women are marginalized. Here again, the question of knowledge is central, since policy documents and guidelines appeal to certain kinds of knowledge. This aspect of our study seeks to offer more than a simple documentation of gaps in education; it aims to explain how institutional policies and procedures are organized, as well as the kinds of actions they authorize – and foreclose. The absence of HIV education initiatives that are relevant to bisexual men and women is to be understood in light of such institutional issues.

This overview of some of the central reasons for the exclusion of bisexuals from HIV research, policy, and education is a necessary background for the development of an alternative, more progressive research agenda. In contrast to the absences outlined above, we develop an empirical investigation of the HIV/STD prevention needs of people who have sexual relations with both men and women. Our project, based in qualitative interviews as well as the creation of educational posters, provides a wealth of empirical data that outline what the problems are, and attempts to intervene in the current situation. The interviews themselves trace a line of fault between the knowledge of everyday people about their HIV/AIDS education needs, and the knowledge advanced within official sites of HIV research, policy, and education. In conclusion, then, we return to this disjuncture. Critical reflection on this line of fault can help us do the work of HIV education differently – arguably, it can ensure that our work is more effective. Our reflections on the lines of fault in knowledge about HIV underlines the importance of institutional ethnography as a framework for critically examining the social and institutional relations of HIV/AIDS prevention in Canada.

Our analysis points to some central splits between how HIV education is organized locally and what people identify as required in this domain. The literal erasure of bisexuality is, of course, one of the central problematics in our study. While the men and women we interview articulate the need for campaigns that address their sexual lives and realities, our analysis of institutions and research considers how bisexuality is made invisible. Current HIV education recognizes only certain populations. Moreover, our study examines the ways in which HIV/AIDS community organizations are central in ensuring which populations and realities are recognized – best illustrated with the argument that this very project is not 'community-based,' since it does not involve the HIV/AIDS establishment agencies. These complicated relations between community organizations, policy, research, and education help us understand how and why the knowledge we have on HIV is circular.

A second line of fault identified in our study is that of gender. Drawing on some work in feminist epidemiology, we consider how mainstream public health minimizes women's specific vulnerabilities to HIV/STD transmission – whether through a complete disregard of women's bodies in the clinical definition of disease, or through establishing a 'hierarchy of transmission' in which matters that are specific to women may be overlooked (ACT-UP/NY 1990; Treichler 1988). The limitations of such an approach are evident when one listens to the voices of the women we interviewed. They tell us about the ways that HIV education and services continue to ignore women's needs – evidenced, for example, in the women who were given HIV education that did not even consider women's bodies, or the women who were refused STD testing, having been told that they were not at risk for STDs since they were sexually involved with other women. These empirical data remind us of the consequences of epidemiological studies that are gendered: women's specific realities remain obscure, and women cannot access the information and services they require.

The absence of HIV/STD education directed to a mainstream audience constitutes a third line of fault identified in our study. Our reflection on policy considers how funding for HIV programs gives priority to certain communities in particular – those already recognized as affected by the HIV/AIDS epidemic. This analysis is in contrast to the needs articulated by the participants in our study, who want to see HIV/AIDS education that is targeted to a mainstream audience. The disjuncture here – between the institutional organization of HIV/AIDS education and the specific needs identified by everyday people – offers a different way to think about how to respond to HIV/AIDS. Instead of a *reactive* response, in which education privileges communities in which HIV rates are already high, our interviewees suggest that HIV education should be organized more proactively, targeting precisely those people who might see themselves as beyond risk, since they are not members of specific communities closely associated with HIV/AIDS in the popular mindset.

These lines of fault, then, are useful for helping us think about how we might organize things differently. The creation of our educational materials, outlined in chapter 7, provides some concrete examples of what this might look like. Importantly, it is research itself that has allowed us to identify these disjunctures, as well as to respond to them. Critical social science research – reflected in this project through both institutional ethnography and participatory action research – has a fundamental role to play in helping us understand the structural reasons underlying specific problems (the absence of information and services relevant to men and women with bisexual behaviour), as well as in articulating meaningful actions to improve the current situation (the development of posters). In chapter 1, we examined the ways in which many social scientific studies are themselves determined by the results of mainstream epidemiological research – for instance, that social scientists focus on the behaviour of members of a particular population (such as gay men) where HIV seroprevalence rates are high. Within this logic, mainstream epidemiology offers a snapshot of populations where a disease is located, and social scientists then engage in more detailed data collection on the attitudes and behaviours of different populations (Gould 1993).

The approach offered throughout this book offers a more critical relation between mainstream public health research and social science inquiry. Indeed, we suggest here that rather than having epidemiology determine the nature of social investigations in the field of HIV/AIDS, social science can itself help us to understand the weaknesses of responding to HIV/AIDS strictly within the terms of mainstream public health and epidemiology. As we have seen, epidemiological research is far from neutral, but rather embodies specific ideas about gender, culture, and sexuality. Critical social science can help us unpack such bias, in order to think about what kind of knowledge would then be needed to understand disease otherwise. Our research begins with this kind of endeavour and identifies the importance of speaking with everyday people about their needs. As Eric Mykalovskiy and Lorna Weir (2004) contend, this kind of approach, which situates the patient as a site of evidence, demonstrates the important contribution social scientific inquiry can make to health research.

In addition to this focus on everyday people as a site of evidence, there are additional ways in which the kind of social scientific inquiry we advocate is relevant for critical knowledge and action. In the first instance, our work considers how knowledge itself is embedded in social relations – for example, how popular misconceptions about bisexuality are omnipresent in the research methodology of scientific studies or are used to justify refusal of funding of empirical research on this subject. In refusing to take the scientific knowledge we have of bisexualities at face value, we gain insight into how and why knowledge itself constitutes social relations of sexuality. Whereas mainstream epidemiology reinforces certain clichés about bisexuality, our research seeks to think critically about how knowledge itself is constructed and used.

Moreover, our consideration of specific institutional policies, procedures, and funding guidelines in HIV/AIDS is useful to understand how certain populations achieve recognition within a state apparatus – as well as how some communities remain unnamed and unnoticed. To explain the lack of information relevant to people who have sexual relations with both men and women requires an analysis of how institutions work – the communities identified as important, and the administration of education according to specific priority populations. Our study is useful for understanding gaps in information for bisexual men and women, as well as for examining the virtual absence of HIV education directed to the mainstream. In this regard, while our institutional analysis began with a specific interest in examining the exclusion of people who have sexual relations with both men and women from HIV educational campaigns, the results of our study tell us something important about HIV education more generally: the current organizational structure makes it difficult to do mainstream HIV/AIDS education. Here, then, an institutional analysis of HIV/AIDS bureaucracy offers insight into more than funding for one particular community (bisexual men and women). Institutional ethnography helps us to see how HIV/AIDS education is organized in a broader sense. In this light, critical social science can assist us in seeing beyond the challenges specific to one particular population or community. Our work, then, is to be considered not as a simple plea for funding bisexual-specific programs (although we do recognize the need for integrating bisexual realities within HIV prevention more broadly). Rather, our research raises critical questions about the limits of organizing our response to HIV according to a model of population health. Such a framework actually pre-empts general mainstream education – precisely the kind of campaigns cited as necessary by the men and women we interviewed.

Also with specific regard to institutions, our analysis uncovers the central role played by certain AIDS community organizations in HIV research, policy, funding, and education. The data we present illustrate how such agencies can also be gate-keepers, ensuring that they remain the sole actors in the field of HIV/AIDS. This dynamic is subtle and complex and reflects particular relations between community organizations and the state within a neoliberal context. Here again, social science inquiry can offer a critical research agenda: not merely accepting the established players in a field as the voice of authority, but examining the manner in which only certain actors achieve recognition – as well as the interests at stake. Institutional ethnography is one tradition within critical social science that facilitates analysis of some of these invisible social relations. This framework helps us to understand how the information available within HIV prevention is an effect of how knowledge itself is organized and produced in the field.

Finally, our action research approach offers a specific illustration of how to put the knowledge we gather into action. While documenting the exclusion of bisexual men and women from HIV/AIDS education is important, it is equally necessary to think practically about how such knowledge can be used. The creation of specific educational materials, based on our empirical data, offers a concrete instance of connecting knowledge and action in a dynamic way. Here, critical social science does more than describe a phenomenon. In contrast to many studies in public health, community health, and mainstream sociology, we give more than a detailed empirical overview of the lives of people who have sexual relations with both men and women. Furthermore, our study provides more than an academic analysis of the problems people experience accessing information and services – although such an analysis is important. By incorporating an action research framework within the design of our study, we develop and propose specific solutions to intervene in the current situation. This kind of social scientific inquiry, then, insists that academic research be intimately connected to action itself. The production of knowledge is oriented both inside and outside the university.

To be sure, the terrain covered by this book is broad, spanning epidemiology, sociology, public policy, community organizing, sexuality, and action research. Our analysis undoubtedly contains limitations in each of these substantive fields. Although we may not satisfy all of the expectations of readers coming from the above fields of inquiry, we seek to ask broad questions that are relevant to each of these domains. More generally, we hope we have made the case for a critical investigation of knowledge in our understanding of, and response to, HIV/AIDS.

We began this book – and this research project – with a simple question: why is there virtually no HIV education in Canada for people who have sexual relations with both men and women? The answer to this question, as we have seen, is complex. From epistemology to methodology, from administrative procedures to relations between community organizations and the state, a number of different factors explain how and why people like bisexual men and women are excluded within HIV research, policy, and education. Critical social scientific inquiry can help us better understand how such exclusion is structured and what can be done about it. This connection between knowledge and action, in our view, offers a useful model to consider in our efforts to respond adequately to the challenges raised by HIV/AIDS.

Notes

Introduction

1 There have been some small-scale research studies on bisexualities in Canada and Québec. One study addresses HIV prevention specifically (Médico et al. 2002), while a second research project considers broader questions of health care and health issues for bisexual men and women (Dobinson et al. 2005; OPHA 2003). Also see Engler (2002) for an analysis of bisexual men as a subset of MSM within a large-scale study in Montréal.

1. The Epistemology of Epidemiology: Understanding the Knowledge and Limits of Public Health Research and Education

1 The HIV diagnostic test is not used to screen out HIV-positive refugee claimants in Canada in a general sense: having HIV is not grounds for refusal. That said, the particular state of overall health of an HIV-positive person is relevant, if the state determines that an individual's condition is likely to cause a burden on the public health care system. Thus, individuals who are HIV-positive but in good health can be accepted as refugees and asylum seekers in Canada. For more information on this matter, see Canadian HIV/AIDS Legal Network (2009).

2 In research on MSM through Pubmed, a database dealing specifically with public health and medical issues, 2031 entries are listed with the search term *MSM*. Coincidentally, the program prompts other search words and suggests that one also search with the terms *black MSM* or *African-American MSM*. The category *MSM black* yields 204 results, while the words *MSM Asian* cites only 36 entries. Perhaps more telling, when one searches with

the specific terms *MSM black active*, one can locate twenty-one entries. A request for articles using the terms *MSM Asian active*, however, produces only 1 result.

2. Institutional Ethnography: Understanding the Links between Research, Policy, and Education on HIV/AIDS

1 For a more advanced and thorough discussion of the intellectual influences that inform IE, see the foreword by James Louis Heap, in Campbell and Ann Manicom (1995, ix–xv).
2 Sociologists will recognize here the influence of ethnomethodology in this attention to how social relations are constituted in and through specific documents. For more on this area, see Garfinkel (1967) and Zimmerman (1974).
3 For an overview of Canada's Federal Initiative on HIV/AIDS, see the Public Health Agency of Canada's website, http://www.phac-aspc.gc.ca/aids-sida/fi-if/index-eng.php.
4 *Leading Together* stipulates that bold targets are required in order to motivate action. That said, it also recognizes that in some instances, 'baseline data' may not be available to accurately measure progress and or the achievement of targets (PHAC 2005a, 23).
5 Committee evaluation summary, file 410-2003-0920, Selection Committee 410-20, SSHRC Standard Research Grants Competition.
6 See committee summary, application 6964-15-2002/5400037, Community-Based HIV/AIDS Research Programme, Health Canada.
7 Translations throughout are by the authors, unless noted otherwise.

3. Methods and Methodology: Designing an HIV Prevention Research Project Relevant to People Who Have Sexual Relations with Both Men and Women

1 The term *ethnocultural* is used in Québec to designate, roughly, communities referred to as 'racial and ethnic minorities' within the Anglo-Canadian and Anglo-American (United States) contexts.
2 See Lombardi and Leger (2006) for an evaluation of this campaign.
3 Sholey (1998) offers a good discussion of the methodological challenges in outreach to men who have sex with men who are not gay-identified.
4 A useful and succinct introduction to CBR can be found in the inaugural issue of the *Canadian Journal of Aboriginal HIV/AIDS Community-Based Research*, available online at www.caan.ca.

4. 'The Message Is Ugly, You Know?' Limits of HIV Education in Québec

1 See OPHA (2003) and Dobinson et al. (2005) for some excellent preliminary work in this regard.
2 In addition to Dobison et al. (2005) and the OPHA (2003), see Medico et al. (2002) for some empirical data related to bisexualities and HIV, based on relatively small sample populations.
3 See the evaluation research conducted on this campaign, Lombardi and Leger (2006).

5. 'Cherchez la femme': The Exclusion of Women in HIV Education and Services

1 See the evaluation of our project, file 6964-15-2003/5400054, HIV/AIDS Research Program, 2003–4 competition, Health Canada.
2 We did not have access to this comment when we received the committee feedback. It was only when we made a request to Access to Information, in order to consult all of the documents (individual evaluations as well as committee discussions) that we discovered the opinion of one reviewer of our research team.
3 This need not necessarily be the case, as one study in Canada reveals that almost a third of men who identified themselves as gay to researchers had had sexual relations with a woman in the past year (Myers et al. 1993). In this regard, one could think it appropriate to develop educational initiatives that include women within gay male communities.

6. 'And That's a Big Gap, I Think': Linking HIV/STD Education and Services

1 Field notes based on interviews with swinger club owner, 12 May 2005.
2 Workshop 'On se protège,' Bi Unité Montréal, 4 April 2005, Montréal.
3 Field notes, 4 April 2005.
4 For an overview of the Specific Populations Fund, see PHAC (2006).

7. Connecting Knowledge and Action: Development and Distribution of HIV and STD Prevention Materials

1 See in particular some of the work on bisexuality and HIV carried out at the Fenway Center in Boston (n.d.), the Parisian group Bi'Cause, who produced a booklet on this subject (2004–7), and the German HIV/AIDS pamphlet

Bisexualität ist eine Möglichkeit, produced by Deutsche AIDS Hilfe (available for order from DAH online at http://www.aidshilfe.de/produkte. php?id=4277).

2 The telephone line was answered live for four hours every weekday, from 3–7 pm. This time of day was selected to allow the possibility of people with regular work hours to contact us during the workday (if they did not want to call from home), or else directly from home (after work hours). Moreover, our voicemail message welcomed people leaving their name and number to speak directly with someone if they so desired. That said, we also informed callers that we answered the phone directly Monday–Friday, 3–7 pm. In this manner, we provided a means to reach us for callers who were not comfortable leaving their name and telephone number on our voicemail.

References

ACT-UP New York. 1990. *Women, AIDS and Activism*. Boston: South End Press.

Angelides, Steven. 2001. *A History of Bisexuality*. Chicago: University of Chicago Press.

ASPC (Agence de Santé Public du Canada). 2006. *Relevé de maladies transmissibles au Canada* 32 (15).

Bailey, J.V., C. Farquhar, C. Owen, and P. Mangtani. 2004. 'Sexually Transmitted Infections in Women Who Have Sex with Women.' *Sexually Transmitted Infections* 80: 244–6.

Bannerji, Himani. 1995. 'Beyond the Ruling Category to What Actually Happens: Notes on James Mill's Historiography in the History of British India.' In Campbell and Manicom, *Knowledge, Experience, and Ruling Relations*, 49–64.

– 2000. *The Dark Side of the Nation: Essays on Multiculturalism, Nationalism and Gender*. Toronto: Canadian Scholars' Press.

Bauer, Greta R., and Seth L. Welles. 2001. 'Beyond Assumptions of Negligible Risk: Sexually Transmitted Diseases and Women Who Have Sex with Women.' *American Journal of Public Health* 91 (8): 1282–6.

Beeker, C. 1993. *A Final Report on Hispanic Nongay-Identified Men Who Have Sex with Other Men: A Formative Research Study*. Atlanta: Center for Disease Control.

Bevier, P.J., M.A. Chiasson, R.T. Heffernan, and K.G. Castro. 1995. 'Women at a Sexually Transmitted Disease Clinic Who Reported Same-Sex Contact: Their HIV Seroprevalence and Risk Behaviors.' *American Journal of Public Health* 85 (10): 1366–71.

Bi'Cause. 2004–7. *Fêter le corps et continuer à vivre*. http://www.pelnet.com/bicause/html/doc/brochure.htm.

Boykin, Keith. 2004. *Beyond the Down Low: Sex, Lies and Denial in Black America*. New York: Carroll and Graf.

Campbell, Marie, and Frances Gregor. 2002. *Mapping Social Relations: A Primer in Doing Institutional Ethnography*. Aurora, ON: Garamond.

Campbell, Marie, and Ann Manicom, eds. 1995. *Knowledge, Experience, and Ruling Relations: Studies in the Social Organization of Knowledge*. Toronto: University of Toronto Press.

Canadian HIV/AIDS Legal Network. 2009. *Canada's Immigration Policy as It Affects People Living with HIV/AIDS: Questions and Answers*. Toronto: Canadian HIV/AIDS Legal Network. http://www.aidslaw.ca/publications/publicationsdocEN.php?ref=97.

CPHA (Canadian Public Health Association). 2005. *Leading Together: Canada Takes Action on HIV/AIDS (2005–2010)*. Ottawa: CPHA.

Crichlow, Wesley. 2004. *Buller Men and Batty Bwoys: Hidden Men in Toronto and Halifax Black Communities*. Toronto: University of Toronto Press.

Deutsche AIDS Hilfe. 2000. *Bisexualität ist eine Möglichkeit*. http://www.aidshilfe.de/produkte.php?id=4277.

Dobinson, Cheryl, with Judy MacDonnell, Elaine Hampson, Jean Clipsham, and Kathy Chow. 2005. 'Improving Access and Quality of Public Health Services for Bisexuals.' *Journal of Bisexuality* 5 (1): 41–78.

EKOS Research Associates. 2003. *HIV/AIDS: An Attitudinal Survey*.

Engler, Kim. 2002. *A Bi-Dimensional Perspective of Men Who Have Sex with Men in the OMEGA Cohort: Bisexualities and Their Sexological and Psychosocial Implications*. MA thesis, Université du Québec à Montréal.

Epstein, Steven. 1996. *Impure Science: AIDS, Activism, and the Politics of Knowledge*. Los Angeles: University of California Press.

Farajajé-Jones, Elias. 1995. 'Fluid Desire: Race, HIV/AIDS, and Bisexual Politics.' In *Bisexual Politics: Theories, Queries, and Visions*, ed. Naomi Tucker, with Liz Highleyman and Rebecca Kaplan, 119–30. New York: Harrington Park Press.

Feldhorst, Anja, ed. 1998. *Bisexualitäten*. Berlin: Deustch AIDS Hilfe.

Fenway Health. n.d. Safer Sex for Bisexuals and Their Partners. http://www.fenwayhealth.org/site/DocServer/safersexbi.pdf?docID=322.

Fung, Richard. 1991. 'Looking for My Penis: The Eroticized Asian in Gay Porn.' In *How Do I Look? Queer Film and Video*, ed. Bad Object Choices, 145–68. Seattle: Bay Press.

Gagnon, M., J.D. Jacob, and D. Holmes. 2010. 'Governing through (In)security: A Critical Analysis of Fear-Based Public Health Campaigns.' *Critical Public Health* 20 (2): 245–56.

Garfinkel, Harold. 1967. *Studies in Ethnomethodology*. Englewood Cliffs, NH: Prentice-Hall.

Gonzales, V., K.M. Washienko, M.R. Krone, L.I. Chapman, E.M. Arredondo, H.J. Huckeba, and A. Downer. 1999. 'Sexual and Drug-Use Risk Factors for HIV and STDs: A Comparison of Women with and without Bisexual Experiences.' *American Journal of Public Health* 89 (12): 1841–6.

Gooß, Ulrich. 2002. *Sexualwissenschaftliche Konzepte der Bisexualität von Männern.* Giessen, Germany: Psychosozial-Verlag.

Gorna, Robin. 1996. *Vamps, Virgins and Victims: How Can Women Fight AIDS?* London: Cassell.

Gould, Peter. 1993. *The Slow Plague: A Geography of the AIDS Pandemic.* Oxford, UK: Blackwell.

Hall, Donald, and Maria Pramaggiore, eds. 1996. *RePresenting Bisexualities: Subjects and Cultures of Fluid Desire.* New York: Routledge.

Hamel, Jean. 2003. *L'échangisme: Un phénomène de société.* Montréal: Éditions CÉQSC.

Heap, James Louis. 1995. 'Foreword.' In Campbell and Manicom, *Knowledge, Experience, and Ruling Relations,* ix–xv.

Herr, Kathryn, and Gary Anderson. 2005. *The Action Research Dissertation: A Guide for Students and Faculty.* Thousand Oaks, CA: Sage.

Honnens, Brigitte. 1998. 'Partnerinnen Bisexueller Männer.' In *Bisexualitäten,* ed. Anja Feldhorst, 81–91. Berlin: Deustch AIDS Hilfe.

Hutchins, Loraine, and Lani Ka'ahumanu. 1991. *Bi Any Other Name: Bisexual People Speak Out.* Boston: Alyson.

Inhorn, Marcia, and K. Lisa Whittle. 2001. 'Feminism Meets the "New" Epidemiologies: Toward an Appraisal of Antifeminist Bias in Epidemiological Research on Women's Health.' *Social Science and Medicine* 53: 553–67.

ISQ. Institut de la statistique du Québec. 1998. *Enquête sociale et de santé 1998.* 2nd ed. Québec: Gouvernement du Québec.

Jette, Christian. 2008. *Les organismes communautaires et la transformation de l'État-providence. Trois décennies de construction de politiques publiques dans le domaine de la santé et des services sociaux.* Québec: Presses de l'université du Québec.

Kalichman, S., R. Roffman, J. Picciano, and M. Bolan. 1998. 'Risk for HIV Infection among Bisexual Men Seeking HIV-Prevention Services and Risks Posed to Their Female Partners.' *Health Psychology* 17: 320–7.

Kennedy, Meagan, and Lynda Doll. 2001. 'Male Bisexuality and HIV Risk.' *Journal of Bisexuality* 1 (2–3): 111–35.

Kinsman, Gary. 1992. 'Managing AIDS Organizing: "Consultation," "Partnership," and the National AIDS Strategy.' In *Organizing Dissent: Contemporary Social Movements in Theory and Practice,* ed. William Carroll, 215–31. Toronto: Garamond.

Kompentenznetz. http://www.kompetenznetz-hiv.de.

Kulick, Don. 1998. *Travesti : Sex, Gender and Culture among Brazilian Transgendered Prostitutes.* Chicago: University of Chicago Press.

Kwakwa, Helena A., and M.W. Ghobrial. 2003. 'Female-to-Female Transmission of Human Immunodeficiency Virus.' *Clinical Infectious Diseases* 36: e40–e41.

Lamoureux, Henri. 2007. *L'action communautaire. Des pratiques en quête de sens.* Montréal: VLB.

Lavoie, René. 1998. 'Deux solitudes: les organismes sida et le communauté gaie.' Dans *Sortir de l'ombre: histoires des communautés lesbienne et gaie de Montréal*, ed. Irène Demczuk and Frank W. Remiggi, 337–62. Montréal: VLB.

Lee, Raymond. 1993. *Doing Research on Sensitive Topics.* London: Sage.

Le Goff, Frédérique, Christopher McAll, and Catherine Montgomery. 2005. *La transformation du communautaire: Expériences d'intervention auprès des jeunes sans-emploi.* Montréal: Éditions Saint-Martin.

Lombardi, A., and Yves Leger. 2006. 'Thinking about "Think Again" in Canada: Assessing an HIV/AIDS Prevention Social Marketing Campaign.' Conference poster presentation, Canadian HIV/AIDS Research Association, Québec City, 25–8 May.

Marrazzo, Jeanne M., Patricia Coffey, and Allison Bingham. 2005. 'Sexual Practices, Risk Perception and Knowledge of Sexually Transmitted Disease Risk among Lesbian and Bisexual Women.' *Perspectives on Sexual and Reproductive Health* 37 (1): 6–12.

Massé, Raymond. 1995. *Culture et santé publique. Les contributions de l'anthropologie à la prévention et à la promotion de la santé.* Montréal: Gaëtan Morin.

Medico, Denise, Joseph Josy Lévy, Joanne Otis, Pierette Laroche, and René Lavoie. 2002. 'La prévention du VIH/sida chez les hommes bisexuels: entre pulsion et confiance.' *Vulnérabilités et prévention VIH/Sida. Enjeux contemporains*, ed. Gaston Godin, Joseph Josy-Lévy, Germain Trottier, in collaboration with Hélène Gagnon, 144–58. Québec: Presses universitaires de l'université Laval.

Mendès-Leité, Rommel. 1996. *Bisexualité: Le dernier tabou.* Paris: Calmann-Lévy.

Miller, Marshall. 2002. '"Ethically Questionable?" Popular Media Reports on Bisexual Men and AIDS.' *Journal of Bisexuality* 2 (1): 93–112.

Mort, Maggie, and Andrew Smith. 2009. 'Beyond Information: Intimate Relations in Sociotechnical Practice.' *Sociology* 43: 215–31.

Myers, Ted, Gaston Godin, Liviana Calzacara, Jean Lambert, and David Locker. 1993. *Au masculin: L'enquête canadienne sur l'infection à VIH menée auprès des hommes gais et bisexuels.* Ottawa: Société canadienne du Sida.

Mykalovskiy, Eric, and Roy Cain. 2008. 'Critical Work: Invigorating Critical Social Science and Humanities Research on HIV/AIDS in Ontario.' Unpublished.

Mykhalovskiy, E., and L. McCoy. 2002. 'Troubling Ruling Discourses of Health: Using Institutional Ethnography in Community-Based Research.' *Critical Public Health* 12 (1): 17–37.

Mykhalovskiy, E., S. Patten, C. Sanders, M. Bailey, and D. Taylor. 2009. 'Beyond Buzzwords: Towards a Community-Based Model of the Integration of HIV Treatment and Prevention.' *AIDS Care* 21 (1): 25–30.

Mykhalovskiy, E., and L. Weir. 2004. 'The Problem of Evidence-Based Medicine: Directions for Social Science.' *Social Science and Medicine* 59 (5): 1059–69.

Namaste, Viviane. 1998. 'The Everyday Bisexual as Problematic: Research Methods beyond Monosexism.' In *Sexualities and Social Action: Inside the Academy and Out*, ed. Janice Ristock and Catherine Taylor, 111–36. Toronto: University of Toronto Press.

Namaste, Viviane, T.H. Vulov, Nada Saghie, Joseph Jean-Gilles, M. Lafrenière, Nancy Leclerc, M. Leroux, Andréa Monette, and R. Williamson. 2007. 'HIV and STD Preventions Needs of Bisexual Women: Results from Projet Polyvalence.' *Canadian Journal of Communication* 32: 357–84.

Naples, Nancy. 2003. *Feminism and Method: Ethnography, Discourse Analysis and Activist Research*. New York: Routledge.

Ng, Roxana. 1988. *The Politics of Community Services: Immigrant Women, Class and the State*. Toronto: Garamond.

– 1995. 'Multiculturalism as Ideology: A Textual Analysis.' In *Knowledge, Experience, and Ruling Relations: Studies in the Social Organization of Knowledge*, ed. Marie Campbell, Ann Manicom, 35–48. Toronto: University of Toronto Press.

OPHA (Ontario Public Health Association). 2003. 'Improving the Access and Quality of Public Health Services for Bisexuals.' Position paper, Toronto.

Orsini, Michael. 2006. 'From "Community Run" to "Community Based"? Exploring the Dynamics of Civil Society–State Transformation in Urban Montréal.' *Canadian Journal of Urban Research* 15 (1): 22–41.

Padian, N., L. Marquis, D. Francis, R. Anderson, G. Rutherford, P. O'Malley, and W. Winkelstein. 1987. 'Male-to-Female Transmission of Human Immunodeficiency Virus.' *Journal of the American Medical Association* 258: 788–90.

Pallota-Chiarolli, Maria. 1998. *Cultural Diversity and Men Who Have Sex with Men: A Review of the Issues, Strategies and Resources*. Melbourne, Australia: National Centre in HIV Research.

Panet Raymond, Jean. 1994. 'Les nouveaux rapports entre l'État et les organismes communautaires à l'ombre de la Loi 120.' *Nouvelles pratiques sociales* 7 (1): 79–83.

Patton, Cindy. 2002. *Globalizing AIDS*. Minneapolis: University of Minnesota Press.

PHAC (Public Health Agency of Canada). 2005. HIV/AIDS Epi Updates. http://www.phac.aspc.gc.ca/publicat/epiu-aepi/epi-05/index-eng.php. Last accessed June 4, 2012.

– HIV/AIDS Policy, Coordination and Programs Division Specific Populations HIV/AIDS Initiative Fund. 2006. http://www.phac-aspc.gc.ca/aids-sida/funding/rfp/rfp06/request0606-eng.php.

Pisani, Elizabeth. 2008. *The Wisdom of Whores: Bureaucrats, Brothels, and the Business of AIDS*. New York: W.W. Norton.

R. v. Labaye. 2005. SCC 80.

Ravet, Jean-Claude. 2009. 'Quel avenir pour l'action communautaire?' http://www.revuerelations.qc.ca/relations/archives/derniers_nos/731/popop/dossier.htm, accessed 13 Nov. 2011.

Reinharz, Shulamit. 1992. *Feminist Methods in Social Research*. New York: Oxford University Press.

Remis, R., and M. Merid. 2004. *The HIV/AIDS Epidemic among Persons from HIV-Endemic Countries in Ontario: Update to December 2002*. Toronto: Department of Public Health Sciences, University of Toronto.

Rich, J.D., A. Back, R.E. Tuomala, and P.H. Kazanjian. 1993. 'Transmission of Human Immunodeficiency Virus Presumed to Have Occurred via Female Homosexual Contact.' *Clinical Infectious Diseases* 17: 1003–5.

Richardson, Denise. 2000. 'The Social Construction of Immunity: HIV Risk Perception and Prevention among Lesbians and Bisexual Women.' *Culture, Health & Sexuality* 2 (1): 33–49.

Rust, Paula. 2000. 'Bisexuality in HIV Research.' In *Bisexuality in the United States: A Social Science Reader*, ed. Paula Rust, 355–99. New York: Columbia University Press.

Scheer, Susan, Ingrid Peterson, Kimberly Page-Shafer, Viva Delgado, A. Gleghorn, J. Ruiz, F. Molitor, W. McFarland, J. Klausner, and the Young Women's Survey Team. 2002. 'Sexual and Drug Use Behavior among Women Who Have Sex with Both Women and Men: Results of a Population-Based Survey.' *American Journal of Public Health* 92 (7): 1110–12.

Scholey, R. 1998. *Delivering HIV Prevention Information to Young Gay and Bisexual Men*. Paper presented at the 12th International Conference on AIDS, Geneva, Switzerland.

Shephard Heim, Benjamin. 1997. *White Nights and Ascending Shadows: An Oral History of the San Francisco AIDS Epidemic*. London: Cassell.

Shilts, Randy. 1987. *And the Band Played On: People, Politics, and the AIDS Epidemic*. New York: St Martin's Press.

Shragge, Eric. 2003. *Activism and Social Change: Lessons for Community and Local Organizing*. Peterborough, ON: Broadview.

SLITSS (Service de Lutte contre les Infections Transmissibles Sexuellement et par le Sang)/MSSS (Ministère de la Santé et des Services Sociaux). 2005. *Portrait des infections transmissibles sexuellement et par le sang (ITSS), de l'hépatite C, de l'infection par le VIH et du sida au Québec*. Québec: SLITSS/MSSS.

Smith, Dorothy. 1987. *The Everyday World as Problematic*. Toronto: University of Toronto Press.

– 2005. *Institutional Ethnography: A Sociology for People*. Walnut Creek, CA: AltaMira Press.

– ed. 2006. *Institutional Ethnography as Practice*. Lanham, MD: Rowman & Littlefield.

Smith, George. 1995. 'Accessing Treatments: Managing the AIDS Epidemic in Ontario.' In Campbell and Manicom, *Knowledge, Experience, and Ruling Relations*, 18–34.

Statistics Canada. 2008. 'Sexual Orientation and Victimization, 2004: Victimization amongst Gays, Lesbians and Bisexuals.' http://www.statcan.gc.ca/pub/85f0033m/85f0033m2008016-eng.htm.

Stevens, Patricia. 1992. 'Lesbian Health Care Research: A Review of the Literature from 1970 to 1990.' *Health Care for Women International* 13 (2): 91–120.

Stevens, Patricia, and Joanne Hall. 2001. 'Sexuality and Safer Sex: The Issues for Lesbians and Bisexual Women.' *Journal of Obstetric, Gynecological, and Neonatal Nursing* (July/August): 439–47.

Stringer, Ernst. 1999. *Action Research*. 2nd ed. Thousand Oaks, CA: Sage.

Tharao, Esther, Notisha Massaquoi, and Senait Teclom. 2006. *Silent Voices of the HIV/AIDS Epidemic: African and Caribbean Women in Toronto, 2002–2004*. Toronto: Women's Health in Women's Hands.

Treichler, Paula. 1988. 'AIDS, Homophobia, and Biomedical Discourse: An Epidemic of Signification.' In *AIDS: Cultural Analysis, Cultural Activism*, ed. Douglas Crimp. Cambridge, MA: MIT Press.

Tripp, Garwood. 1988. 'Fear Advertising: It Doesn't Work!' *Health Promotion* (Winter 1988/9).

Troncosa, A.P., A. Romani, C.M. Carranza, J.R. Macias, and R. Masini. 1995. 'Probable HIV Transmission by Female Homosexual Contact.' *Medicina* 55: 334–6.

Trostle, James. 2005. *Epidemiology and Culture*. New York: Cambridge University Press.

Tucker, Naomi, ed. 1995. *Bisexual Politics: Theories, Queries and Visions*. New York: Harrington.

UNAIDS – United Nations Program on AIDS. 2010. *Report on the Global HIV/AIDS Epidemic, 2008*. Geneva: Joint United Nations Program on AIDS.

White, Deena. 1992. 'La santé et les services sociaux: réforme et remises en question.' In *Le Québec en jeu. Comprendre les grands défies*, ed. Gérard Daigle and Guy Rocher, 225–48. Montréal: Presses universitaires de l'université de Montréal.

Wilgis, Barbara. 2008. 'Sexually Transmitted Infections: An Overview & Update.' Manitoba HIV Conference, Winnipeg, November.

Worth, Heather. 2003. 'The Myth of the Bisexual Infector? HIV Risk and Men Who Have Sex with Men and Women.' *Journal of Bisexuality* 3 (2): 71–92.

Zimmerman, Don. 1974. 'Fact as Practical Accomplishment.' In *Ethnomethodology: Selected Readings*, ed. Roy Turner, 128–43. Markham, ON: Penguin.